An introduction to pharmacovigilance

An introduction to pharmacovigilance

Patrick Waller

Consultant in Pharmacovigilance and Pharmacoepidemiology
Southampton, UK

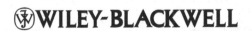

WILEY-BLACKWELL

A John Wiley & Sons, Ltd., Publication

Registered office: John Wiley & Sons Ltd, The Atrium, Southern Gate, Chichester, West Sussex, PO19 8SQ, UK

Editorial offices: 9600 Garsington Road, Oxford, OX4 2DQ, UK

The Atrium, Southern Gate, Chichester, West Sussex, PO19 8SQ, UK

111 River Street, Hoboken, NJ 07030-5774, USA

For details of our global editorial offices, for customer services and for information about how to apply for permission to reuse the copyright material in this book please see our website at www.wiley.com/wiley-blackwell

Library of Congress Cataloging-in-Publication Data

Waller, Patrick

An introduction to pharmacovigilance / by Patrick Waller.

 p. cm.

Includes index.

ISBN: 9781405194716

1. Drugs—Side effects. 2. Pharmacoepidemiology. I. Title. [DNLM:

1. Pharmacoepidemiology—methods. 2. Drug Monitoring—methods. 3. Pharmaceutical Preparations—adverse effects. 4. Pharmaceutical Preparations—standards. QZ 42 W198i 2010]

RM302.5.W35 2010

615'.7042—dc22

2009009656

A catalogue record for this book is available from the British Library.

Set in 9.25/12 pt Meridien Roman by Macmillan Publishing Solutions, Chennai, India

1   2010

The book is dedicated to the memory of the late Dr. Susan M. Wood, an inspirational person who worked tirelessly in the field of pharmacovigilance for 10 years before her premature death in 1998.

Contents

Acknowledgements

I am most grateful to the following people who provided valuable comments on a draft manuscript: Anthony Cox, Stephen Evans, Hilary Pearce, Jakob Petersen and Amarlok Sidhu.

Foreword

No drug which is pharmacologically effective is without hazard. Furthermore not all hazards can be known before a drug is marketed. This was the clear conclusion of the first chairman of the UK's Committee on Safety of Drugs, Derrick Dunlop, in the mid-1970s, and it remains as true today.

Pharmacovigilance, which encompasses the processes involved in identifying, assessing and minimising the risks associated with medicines in clinical use, is now accepted as a vital public health function. As a direct result of the thalidomide tragedy in the 1960s, notification systems for reporting information on adverse drug reactions to the authorities were put in place in most countries.

Since then, the science, methodologies and tools of pharmacovigilance have evolved, largely in response to the growing complexity of drug safety issues. Examples of this complexity include drug-related harms which may be similar to those of the background pathologies in the population treated; harms which may be apparent only in very long-term use; and harms which may be difficult to distinguish from the condition itself being treated.

Evaluating risks as complex as these requires a range of approaches and data sources, and sound judgement in applying them. It is no longer appropriate to talk about moving up a hierarchy of evidence away from less robust forms of data such as single case adverse reaction reports, but of an integrated approach potentially involving a plurality of evidence.

Public expectations have grown too, and delays in acting on drug safety issues are not accepted. Medicines regulators have shifted from a largely reactive response to drug safety issues, to a more proactive approach. Companies and regulators plan safety studies and implement active surveillance to fill in the knowledge gaps that inevitably exist at the time of market authorisation, which is still based on clinical trials designed principally to show a drug's efficacy.

The concept of 'good pharmacovigilance practice' is now widely accepted. But what does this really mean? It must be based on a sound understanding of the key principles – the what and why and how. Even more important, such knowledge needs to be capable of application in less than ideal circumstances, when information is scarce and evidence less robust than desirable.

The published literature on pharmacovigilance is rich in reviews, case studies, criticism and debate, advocacy for particular approaches, and exciting new methodologies. What has been lacking, however, is an overview of the state of knowledge that is clear, comprehensive and accessible. Those embarking on a career in pharmacovigilance or simply wishing to gain a sound working knowledge of the discipline will find what they need to know here in one place.

The challenge of pharmacovigilance today is as great, if not greater, than after the thalidomide tragedy. If the public, patients and health professionals are to be confident in the products they use, it is a challenge worthy of the commitment of all involved in the development, marketing and regulation of medicines.

Dr. June Raine, Director of the Vigilance and Risk Management of Medicines Division, Medicines and Healthcare Products Regulatory Agency, London, UK and Chair of the EU Pharmacovigilance Working Party

Preface

Everyone knows that safety is important but apart from a few people whose job it is to oversee safety, this is probably something that most people have at the back of their minds for most of the time. There are likely to be two reasons for this – firstly, safety is about something adverse not happening (and we tend to be more concerned about things which are happening) and, secondly, it seems to be human nature to think that 'it will not happen to me', perhaps as a mechanism for coping with potential threat of something devastating.

The past decade has seen a marked rise in the numbers of people working in the field of clinical drug safety or pharmacovigilance, mostly in the pharmaceutical industry. The trend seems likely to continue, hopefully reflecting a greater focus on the safety of medicines. This book is specifically targeted at newcomers to the field who, of necessity, are often narrowly focused, and it aims to provide them with a brief and broad introduction to the field. My purpose here is to aid rapid understanding of the environment and key principles of pharmacovigilance at the industry/regulatory interface.

My background is in regulation and my experience is of the UK and EU systems and I readily acknowledge these inherent biases in my narrative. This book probably will not help the newcomers with detailed day-to-day aspects of their job but I hope it will enable them to see where they fit into a bigger picture. I have assumed that readers will at least have a science degree but not necessarily much specific knowledge about drugs.

The new entrant needs to know how we got where we are today. The most important historical drug safety issues have shaped the development of pharmacovigilance and I have therefore used these as a starting point. I hope that the book will also help the newcomers to appreciate that they are now working in an interesting and important field that is likely to develop much in the near future.

I have deliberately not included any reference citations within the text since, initially, I hope the reader will want to read on rather than go elsewhere. Ample references can be found in the larger texts on to which the reader should next move. In the last chapter, I have selectively cited some important sources that might usefully be consulted for further reading. A glossary defining key terms is provided at the end for reference.

Patrick Waller

CHAPTER 1

What is pharmacovigilance and how has it developed?

Origins and definition of pharmacovigilance

In the beginning, there was thalidomide. It can be argued that the history of pharmacovigilance goes back further but, for practical purposes, the story of modern pharmacovigilance begins there.

In the late 1950s there was little, if any, regulation of medicines outside the USA (where thalidomide was not marketed), and their testing and development was almost entirely in the hands of pharmaceutical companies. In the case of thalidomide, unjustified claims of safety in pregnancy were made and its use as a sedative was targeted at pregnant women. The drug turned out to be a teratogen, producing a variety of birth defects but particularly limb defects known as phocomelia (see Figure 1.1). Worldwide, about 10,000 fetuses were affected, particularly in Germany where the drug was first marketed. Since phocomelia was otherwise a very rare congenital abnormality, the existence of a major increase in its incidence did not go unnoticed in Germany but the cause was initially thought to be environmental. In 1961 a series of just three cases associated with thalidomide was reported in *The Lancet*, the problem was finally recognised and the drug withdrawn from sale.

At the beginning of the 1960s, publication of possible adverse effects of drugs in the medical literature was effectively the only mechanism for drawing attention to them. Thalidomide produced a non-lethal but visible and shocking adverse effect, leading people to ask why so many damaged babies had been born before anything had been done? This question is central to subsequent

An Introduction to Pharmacovigilance. By Patrick Waller.
Published 2010 by Blackwell Publishing, ISBN: 978-1-4051-9471-6.

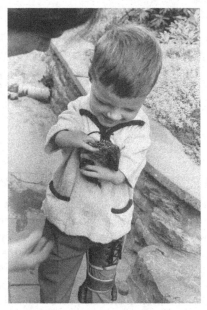

Figure 1.1 Child affected by thalidomide-induced phocomelia.

developments. It is unlikely that we will ever be able to predict and prevent all the harms which may be caused by medicines but limiting the damage to much smaller numbers is now achievable. Today we would expect to be able to identify an association between drug and outcome analogous to thalidomide and phocomelia after the occurrence of less than 10 cases, i.e. at least three orders of magnitude more effectively than five decades ago.

The overriding lesson learnt from thalidomide was that we cannot just wait until a drug safety problem, quite literally in this case, hits us between the eyes. So thalidomide led directly to the initial development of the systems we now have, although it is only quite recently (i.e. since the early 1990s) that the term pharmacovigilance has become widely accepted.

Pharmacovigilance has been defined by the WHO as '*The science and activities relating to the detection, assessment, understanding and prevention of adverse effects or any other drug-related problems*'. There are other definitions but this very broad one seems to be the most appropriate since there is a clear implication that the process is one of 'risk management'. This is a concept which is applicable to many aspects of modern life but, surprisingly, its explicit use in relation to pharmaceuticals is quite a recent development.

Thalidomide is not merely of historical interest since in the last few years it has made something of a comeback. The reasons for this exemplify the point about risk management since the risk of fetal malformation can be successfully managed by avoidance of the drug during pregnancy. It also demonstrates another concept which is central to the practice of pharmacovigilance – the balance of benefit and risk. Thalidomide appears to have benefits in some diseases that are otherwise difficult to treat conditions, e.g. refractory multiple myeloma – these appear to outweigh the risk of fetal malformation if there is an effective pregnancy prevention scheme in place. A further point which thalidomide illustrates well, and is relevant to many other drug safety issues, is that not everyone is at the same risk of a particular adverse effect. In this case, a substantial part of the population i.e. women who are not of childbearing capacity, are not at risk at all.

Main lessons from thalidomide

• The need for adequate testing of medicines prior to marketing.
• The need for government regulation of medicines.
• The need for systems to *identify* the adverse effects of medicines.
• The potential relationship between marketing claims and safety.
• Avoidance of unnecessary use of medicines in pregnancy.
• That some risks can be successfully minimised.

The ramifications of the thalidomide tragedy were many-fold but the key lesson for the development of pharmacovigilance was that active systems for detecting hazards are needed. Within a few years this had been taken forward with the introduction of voluntary (or 'spontaneous') schemes for reporting of suspected adverse drug reactions (ADRs). These have stood the test of time as an alerting mechanism or 'early warning system' and will be covered in more detail in Chapter 3.

Scope and purposes of pharmacovigilance

In the past, the process of pharmacovigilance has often been considered to start when a drug is authorised for use in ordinary practice. Nowadays, it is more commonly considered to include all safety-related activity beyond the point at which humans are first exposed to a new medicinal drug.

The ultimate purpose of pharmacovigilance is to minimise, in practice, the potential for harm that is associated with all active medicines. Although data about all types of ADRs are collected, the main focus is on identifying and preventing those which are defined to be *serious*. This means an ADR which meets at least one of the following criteria:

- Fatal
- Life-threatening
- Causes or prolongs hospitalisation
- Results in long-term disability

Additionally, all congenital abnormalities are considered serious and the definition of 'serious' allows the application of medical judgement such that a reaction may be considered serious, even if there is not clear evidence that one of the above criteria is met.

Non-serious reactions are important to individual patients and health professionals involved in their treatment but they can usually be managed clinically and they impact much less on the balance of benefit of risk and the public health. Thus, pharmacovigilance may be seen as a public health function in which reductions in the occurrence of serious harms are achievable through measures which promote the safest possible use of medicines and/or provide specific safeguards against known hazards. Pregnancy prevention in users of thalidomide is an example of such a safeguard; monitoring white blood cell counts to detect agranulocytosis (absent white blood cells) in users of the antipsychotic drug clozapine is another.

In order to minimise harms there is first a need to identify and assess the impact of unexpected potential hazards. For most medicines, serious ADRs are rare; otherwise their detection would result in the drug not reaching or being withdrawn from the market. For products which do reach the market, serious hazards are seldom identified during pre-marketing clinical trials because sample sizes are almost invariably too small to detect them. In addition, the prevailing conditions of clinical trials – selected patients, short durations of treatment, close monitoring and specialist supervision – almost invariably mean that they will underestimate the frequency of ADRs relative to what will really occur in ordinary practice.

During pre-marketing clinical development, the aims of pharmacovigilance are rather different to the broad public health function described above. In volunteer studies and clinical trials there is an overriding need to protect individuals being exposed. There is also a need to gather information on harms which occur in order to make a provisional assessment of safety and to plan for post-marketing safety development.

Development of pharmacovigilance since the 1960s

In the early 1970s another drug safety disaster occurred – this was the multi-system disorder known as the oculo-mucocutaneous syndrome caused by practolol (Eraldin) – a cardioselective beta-blocker used to treat angina and hypertension. As in the case of thalidomide, several thousand individuals were permanently damaged before the association was recognised. The fundamental problem in this instance was a failure of timely identification despite having an early warning system in place. Ultimately the system was dependent on doctors suspecting an association between drug and disease. Probably because of the unusual nature of the syndrome – dry eyes, skin rash and bowel obstruction – and a long latency period (averaging almost two years in respect of the onset of the most serious bowel manifestations), relevant cases were not reported until the association was identified in the medical literature. Around 3,000 cases were then retrospectively reported to the UK 'Yellow Card' scheme, an example of the potential effect of publicity on ADR reporting. Subsequent attempts to develop an animal model of practolol toxicity failed, indicating that the problem could not have been predicted from pre-clinical studies.

Main lessons from practolol
- Some adverse effects are not predictable from pre-clinical studies.
- Spontaneous reporting schemes are not invariably effective.
- Long latency effects and clinical manifestations not known to be related to other drugs may not be suspected as ADRs by doctors.
- Additional, more systematic methods of studying post-marketing safety are needed.

The overriding message from practolol was that spontaneous ADR reporting alone is insufficient as a means of studying post-marketing safety. Thus, in the late 1970s various schemes designed to closely monitor the introduction of new drugs were suggested, but most of them were not implemented. The basic idea was that initial users of new drugs would be identified through prescriptions and monitored systematically rather than waiting for someone to recognise a possible adverse effect. The concept did come to fruition in the UK in the early 1980s with the development of 'prescription-event monitoring', a method which is still in use today (see Chapter 3).

The first drug studied by prescription-event monitoring was benoxaprofen (Opren), a non-steroidal anti-inflammatory drug (NSAID) which frequently produced photosensitivity reactions, i.e. rashes in light-exposed areas. A published case series of five deaths related to hepatic and renal failure led to withdrawal of the drug in 1982, even though some doubts were expressed as to whether they were caused by the drug, particularly as prescription-event monitoring did not reveal any indication of these effects. Many of the patients who experienced serious ADRs with benoxaprofen were elderly; this was due to reduced excretion of the drug as a consequence of renal impairment. Even though it is well-recognised that many patients who use NSAIDs are elderly, benoxaprofen had not been adequately studied in this population prior to marketing. A reduction in the dosage recommendations for the elderly was implemented briefly but it was too late to save the drug. Because the usage of benoxaprofen took off rapidly after launch and an important adverse effect – photosensitivity reactions – was common, a large number of spontaneous reports were received in a short period of time, swamping the primitive computer systems then used and pointing up the need for purpose-designed databases. The issue also illustrated the need for patients to be properly informed about possible ADRs and how to minimise the risk – in this case by avoiding exposure to the sun. It was therefore influential in moving us towards the introduction of patient information leaflets – these became compulsory in the EU during the 1990s.

Main lessons from benoxaprofen

- Uncertainty about cause and effect from individual case reports – further impetus to the need for formal post-marketing studies.
- The need to study a drug in the population that will use it (e.g. the elderly).
- The need for purpose-designed computer systems to handle ADRs more promptly and effectively.
- The concept of intensive surveillance of new drugs, achieved in the UK by the introduction of the Black Triangle scheme (see Glossary).
- The need for patients to be informed about possible ADRs.

As it turned out, benoxaprofen was just the first of a series of NSAIDs withdrawn for various safety reasons in the 1980s. During this decade, pharmaceutical companies started to conduct their own post-marketing surveillance studies and UK guidelines related to their conduct were drawn up in 1987. However, initially, the value of such studies turned out to be limited because they usually lacked comparator groups and often failed to meet the planned sample-size. The UK guidelines were revised in 1993 with the aim of improving the quality of studies. The principles of the revised, so-called Safety Assessment of Marketed Medicines or SAMM, guidelines also became a blueprint for the first EU level guidance on the topic.

During the mid-1980s, the term pharmacoepidemiology was first used to mean the scientific discipline of the study of drug use and safety at a population level. The discipline developed strongly during the 1990s with the increasing use of computerised databases containing records of prescriptions and clinical outcomes for rapid and efficient study of potential safety hazards. In some instances prescription records are held in a separate database to clinical events, and linkage between the two databases needs to be achieved through some common identifier in the two sets of data in order to study adverse events at an individual patient level.

Towards the end of the 1980s pharmacovigilance eventually recognised and started to deal with the problem of dependence on benzodiazepines – so-called 'minor tranquillisers' such as chlordiazepoxide (Librium) and diazepam (Valium) that had been introduced in the 1960s. Advice was issued to limit the dose and duration of such treatments although, even today, such recommendations are widely ignored. The issue brought into focus the problems faced in dealing with the misuse and abuse of prescription drugs. This is another example of a situation where spontaneous ADR reporting failed to highlight an important concern, the issue eventually coming into focus as a result of pressure from advocates for groups of affected patients.

As well as the problem of delayed identification of real hazards, pharmacovigilance has suffered from the reverse, i.e. apparent identification of hazards which turn out not to be real. To some extent this is inherent in a system which relies much on clinical suspicions – sometimes these will be wrong. The consequences are that sometimes a drug may be unnecessarily withdrawn or people become too scared to use it. For example, Debendox (or Bendectin), a combination product containing an antihistamine doxylamine, was widely used for the treatment of nausea and vomiting in pregnancy in the 1970s. It was withdrawn in the early 1980s on the basis of concerns that it might cause fetal malformations, a concerted campaign against the drug and impending litigation. At the time, the evidence of a hazard was very weak but it was not possible to exclude a significant risk to the fetus. Subsequently, many studies of this potential association were performed and collectively they provided no evidence of an increased risk of fetal malformations. This example illustrates the intrinsic difficulty of disproving the existence of a hazard once concern has been raised. A more recent, very high profile example illustrating the same point was the suggestion made in late 1990s that combined measles, mumps and rubella (MMR) vaccine might be a cause of autism in children. Despite there being little credible evidence for this suggestion, it was impossible to completely disprove it and hard to convince worried parents. Vaccine campaigns were damaged and a significant number of cases of measles occurred in the UK for the first time in many years.

The mother of all drug safety scares occurred with oral contraceptives (OCs) in 1995. It was not the first 'pill' scare – this story began in the late 1960s when it was discovered through spontaneous ADR reporting and confirmed in formal studies that combined OCs (containing an oestrogen and a progestagen) increased the risk of venous thromboembolism (VTE). This led to a reduction in the dose of oestrogen to 20–30μg of ethinyloestradiol which lessened (but did not abolish) the risk without compromising efficacy. Nevertheless, when the risk of thrombosis became public knowledge many women were scared and stopped taking OCs. It is important to recognise that most women using OCs are relatively young and healthy – this impacts considerably on their perception of the risk. When OCs are stopped abruptly by sexually active women without immediate use of an effective alternative, unwanted pregnancies occur and abortion rates increase. The have been several 'pill' scares over the years related to VTE and also to other safety issues – e.g. a possible association with myocardial infarction and a small increase in the risk of breast cancer. In each instance, many women who stopped using OCs later returned to using OCs but the public health impact of each of these scares in terms of unwanted pregnancies was considerable. This has been particularly unfortunate since pregnancy itself is fundamentally riskier than using any OC and there may also be compensating health benefits from using them.

In 1995 a WHO study of OCs unexpectedly found a two-fold increase in the risk of VTE when use of so-called 'third-generation' (3G) OCs was compared to 'second-generation' (2G) OCs. The difference between these pills was the progestagen component – desogestrel or gestodene for 3G OCs and levonorgestrel for 2G OCs. This was surprising as it had always been considered that VTE risk was simply related to the dose of the oestrogen component of the pill. Another multinational study which could address the relative safety of 3G and 2G OCs was ongoing and a further study was quickly conducted using a UK database. Within about three months the results of three studies were available and their findings were all quite similar. Arguments were put forward that the associations seen in these studies were not necessarily causal and also that it was possible that 3G OCs might have benefits which would compensate for the increase in VTE risk. There was general agreement that the absolute level of risk – VTE is quite rare in healthy young women, even if they take the pill – was not such that 3G OCs should be withdrawn from the market but nevertheless the UK's expert regulatory committee felt that doctors and women needed to know. Despite a clear message being provided that no one should stop taking OCs, many women did, presumably because the media coverage scared them. It did not help that the principal investigator of one of the studies flew from Canada to London to give a press conference criticising the committee's advice because the public get more worried when experts disagree. At the time, the European Medicines Agency had recently been formed but co-operation on nationally authorised products was in its infancy. Various authorities in Europe and around the world adopted different positions and it was not until 2001 that the EU reached an agreed position on the issue.

Over a period of several years, more studies were done and the effects of the various progestagens on blood clotting investigated. Ultimately, it was shown that there were plausible differential effects of these agents on clotting and there was enough consistency in the risk data to convince most scientists that the observed association was causal. But, despite good intentions all round, it was hard to escape the feeling that more harm than good had been done and that the communication tools used were inadequate. In 1997 the WHO convened a meeting of experts to specifically consider how communication in pharmacovigilance could be improved (see Chapter 5).

Main lessons learned from the OC safety issues
- Drugs are sometimes marketed at the wrong dose.
- There may be differences in safety between drugs of the same class.
- Harm may result from safety warnings.
- Uncertainty and debate about risks may fuel public concern.
- The power of the media to influence users is much greater than the authorities.
- The need for greater international co-operation in pharmacovigilance.
- There is a need to develop more effective communication tools.

One important point about the OC issues discussed above is that the data on which they were based did not (after the initial signal in the 1960s) come from spontaneous ADR reporting. Despite that, causation was debatable because the studies were not randomised trials but 'observational'. VTE is a sufficiently rare outcome in young women that it would be extremely difficult to conduct a large enough clinical trial to detect a doubling of risk.

Later in life, women have also been prescribed female sex hormones – in lower doses and as replacement therapy (HRT). In this age group the baseline risks of VTE, arterial cardiovascular disease and various cancers are much greater and therefore, it is more feasible to study them in clinical trials although they do need to be large and long-term. Therefore observational studies of these outcomes were performed first and, in general, they appeared to show that HRT *reduced* the risk of arterial disease outcomes, i.e. myocardial infarction and stroke. HRT was not authorised for the purpose of reducing cardiovascular risk but in the 1980s and 1990s it was quite widely used for this purpose. The fundamental problem in performing such studies is that women using HRT may be healthier to start with, although it is possible to address this, at least to some extent, in the design and analysis. Another important point is that the outcome in question is a *benefit* (i.e. a reduction in risk) and, because of such biases, observational studies rarely provide convincing evidence of benefit. It is generally accepted that randomised trials are needed to establish efficacy and benefit.

Eventually, large randomised trials were set up but they had to be stopped early because they tended to show the opposite of what was expected – i.e., an increase in cardiovascular risk. Warnings were issued and, because there is no major downside to suddenly stopping HRT, communication was intrinsically easier than with OCs. Indeed, the intended effect of the warnings was that women who were inappropriately using long-term HRT should stop taking it. However, conveying the right messages was not straightforward because there were multiple risks involved, and they are time-dependent and cannot simply be expressed as a proportion (e.g. 1 in 100).

HRT, like the last two issues I am going to cover here, came to a critical point in the first three or four years of the new millennium. However, history is not yet 'complete' on any of these issues, indeed one often wonders whether it ever can be – e.g. with the return of previously withdrawn drugs like thalidomide and clozapine. The latter is an antipsychotic drug which was first introduced in the 1970s and then withdrawn following reports of agranulocytosis, i.e. absence of white blood cells. It was reintroduced with compulsory blood monitoring around 1990.

Selective serotonin re-uptake inhibitors (SSRIs) are antidepressants which were brought to the market in the late 1980s and have since largely replaced older, 'tricyclic' antidepressants such as amitriptyline. The main reason why they have done so – apart from effective marketing – is that they are less toxic to the heart in overdose, i.e. there is a greater margin of safety in relation to dose. Depressed patients are at risk of taking an overdose and therefore this is potentially an important advantage.

There have been two controversial issues with SSRIs – withdrawal reactions and a possible increase in the risk of suicide. Problems experienced by patients when they stop treatments are often quite difficult to assess because they could possibly be related to recurrence of the disease. Nevertheless, the potential for SSRIs to produce withdrawal reactions was identified during their development, and when spontaneous reports were received post-marketing it was hardly a new 'signal'. There were very large numbers of such reports received but few were serious and the level of usage of the drugs was high. Over a period of years it became clear that the problem was occurring much more commonly than initially thought, particularly in users of paroxetine (Seroxat), a fairly short-acting drug. Ultimately, greater care was needed in withdrawing patients more gradually from these drugs. Suggestions have been made that SSRIs are drugs of dependence but most scientists do not accept this because features such as craving and dose-escalation are generally absent. Importantly, it emerged that the nature of some of the more unpleasant symptoms patients experienced – e.g. so-called 'electric shock' sensations in the head was being lost in the data processing systems. This was due to inadequate coding such cases often became 'paraesthesia', something that hardly conveys how unpleasant such sensations can be. Thus it was recognised that we need better ways to capture unusual patient experiences and this gave considerable impetus to allowing patients to report their adverse reactions to the authorities. That approach had been used in the USA for many years but hardly at all in Europe until the early years of the new millennium.

The possibility that any drug might increase the risk of an outcome associated with the disease it is being used to treat is invariably difficult to evaluate. Suicidal feelings and actions are relatively common in depressed patients and it is not surprising when they occur in a patient who has recently started treatment. Nevertheless, around 1990 a clinician in the USA saw several patients treated with fluoxetine (Prozac) who had suicidal thoughts and he published a case series suggesting that the drug might be responsible. This prompted a review of all the clinical trial data for the drug which did not support the proposition but it was never completely refuted. Over the years more clinical trial data accumulated for various drugs in the class and studies were conducted in children and adolescents, the latter being a high-risk group for suicide. Even in severely depressed patients, completed suicides are rare in clinical trials and therefore the evidence that is available relates mostly to attempted suicide (also uncommon in trials) and thoughts of suicide measured on various scales. Trials of paroxetine in children produced some potentially worrying findings that for some time were known only to the manufacturer. When the regulatory authorities eventually received the data, they issued warnings against the use of this drug in children. The company was investigated and prosecution considered but the law was found to be insufficiently clear that they were obliged to immediately submit concerning clinical trial data to the authorities when a trial was being conducted outside the authorised indication. This issue again pointed to the potential importance of clinical trials to the assessment of safety and raised concern about a lack of transparency with clinical trial data. Already, considerable steps have been taken towards making clinical trial data publicly available through mechanisms other than publication in the literature which is slow and selective. The jury is still out on whether SSRIs directly increase the risk of suicide but there is general agreement that the early phase of treatment is a high-risk period and that careful monitoring of patients is required.

Finally, what is probably the most important drug safety issue of recent years? The answer is the increased risk of cardiovascular outcomes associated with selective COX-2 inhibitors (coxibs). This possibility was first uncovered in basic research but not followed through; the first clinical indication of a problem came from a trial known as VIGOR which was published in 2000. At the time, two drugs in the class – rofecoxib and celecoxib – had just been authorised. The VIGOR study was a randomised comparison of rofecoxib and naproxen (a standard NSAID) designed to establish whether or not there was a difference in the rates of serious gastrointestinal adverse effects of these two drugs. In that respect, rofecoxib was clearly preferable and the trial results led to rapid uptake of coxibs – on the basis that they were supposedly safer. The VIGOR study also found an important difference in the rate of cardiovascular events such as myocardial infarction – these were five-fold more common in patients taking rofecoxib, compared to naproxen. This information was included in the original publication but lacked prominence and was presented as a five-fold reduction with naproxen rather than an increase with rofecoxib. The paper has since been the subject of extensive criticism.

Over the years there have been suggestions that standard NSAIDs might reduce the risk of cardiovascular outcomes (as aspirin does) and one explanation for the finding in the VIGOR study put forward was that naproxen is 'cardioprotective' whereas rofecoxib is not. Ultimately, it took a large clinical trial comparing rofecoxib with placebo to establish beyond any doubt that this was an adverse effect of rofecoxib (rather than a lack of benefit) and the findings of that study led to the drug being withdrawn from the market in late 2004. This event sent shockwaves around the world that are still reverberating leading people to question why such a trial had not been done much earlier, i.e. before millions of people had used the drug. It also left a big cloud hanging over the remaining drugs in the class – some have been withdrawn and some remain in the market. At one stage, the proposition that coxibs might be given to people at high risk of gastrointestinal and low risk of cardiovascular disease seemed reasonable but it has since been discovered that, to a considerable extent, risk factors for these problem overlap in individual patients. To make matters even more complicated, it appears that some standard NSAIDs might also increase the risk of cardiovascular events and, at the present time, our ability to assess the relative safety of drugs in the same class remains rather limited.

Main lessons learned from recent major safety issues

- The need for vigorous follow-up of safety signals with appropriate studies.
- The difficulty of assessing outcomes which are related to the drug indication.
- The potential value of clinical trials in assessing safety and the importance of the choice of comparator drug(s).
- Important safety data may emerge from clinical trials performed for other purposes.
- The need for greater openness about clinical trial data.
- The potential importance of off-label use (e.g. in children) to safety.
- There is a need to evaluate medicines properly in children.
- The need for greater patient involvement in drug safety.
- The complexity of evaluating and communicating multiple risks (and benefits).
- The need for regulatory authorities to have powers to ensure that companies adequately investigate potential risks with marketed products.

Conclusion

The issues discussed above are necessarily selective and my narration of them is broad. The intention is primarily to illustrate that pharmacovigilance has experienced many teething problems and that most of its developments have been in response to quite specific lessons learned from landmark safety issues. In this chapter, I have tried to illustrate what pharmacovigilance is and how it has progressed over a period of nearly half a century. Despite that progress, no one should doubt that there is a long way to go yet. The current limitations of the discipline and how we might overcome them are considered in Chapter 8.

CHAPTER 2
Basic concepts

Introduction

The two most important concepts in pharmacovigilance are oppo-
sites, i.e. harm and safety. The usual term for harm related to a
medicine is an adverse drug reaction (ADR). Since pharmacovigilance is fundamentally about preventing ADRs, this concept will
be considered first through a summary of relevant definitions,
classification systems which have been proposed, their nature and
mechanisms, predisposing factors, and the overall public health
burden and costs associated with them. Subsequently, the concept
of safety will be defined and discussed, particularly in the context
of balancing harms with benefits. Finally, I will consider the issue
of causation – how we go about deciding whether or not a patient
has experienced an ADR or whether a drug really is responsible for
an apparent safety problem?

Adverse drug reactions

Definitions
Standard, internationally agreed definitions of side-effect, ADR and
adverse event may be paraphrased as follows:
- A **side-effect** is an *unintended effect of a medicine*. Normally it is
  undesirable but it could be beneficial (e.g. an anxiolytic effect
  from a beta-blocker prescribed for hypertension).
- An **adverse drug reaction (ADR)** is an *unintended and noxious
  effect* that is attributable to a medicine when it has been given
  within the normal range of doses used in man.

An Introduction to Pharmacovigilance. By Patrick Waller.
Published 2010 by Blackwell Publishing, ISBN: 978-1-4051-9471-6.

- An **adverse event (AE)** is an undesirable occurrence that occurs in the context of drug treatment but which *may or may not* be causally related to a medicine.

The difference between an ADR and an AE is crucial and yet these terms are widely misused, particularly within the pharmaceutical industry. In practice, determining whether or not a drug is responsible for a particular AE in an individual patient is often difficult and a judgement has to be made (see below for an explanation of the principles on which this judgement is based). When the judgement of a clinician caring for the patient is that the drug is a possible cause, this should be called a *suspected ADR*. Reports of such suspicions form the basis of spontaneous ADR reporting schemes and the key point about such data is that they are a *subset* of all the AEs occurring during drug treatment which someone, generally a health professional who has seen the patient, has identified as possibly being drug-related. It is the clinician's experience and intuition that enables him or her to suspect a drug as the cause but, of course, that suspicion may or may not be correct.

Use of the term 'AE' properly should imply that a more systematic data collection process has been used so that events will be included regardless of whether or not anyone believes they might be caused by a drug. For example, in most clinical trials it is a standard practice to document all AEs and the best way of determining whether a drug is responsible for a particular type of event from such data is by comparison with a control group. For example, if 10% of patients exposed to an active drug experienced headache compared to 2% on placebo then this is an estimate that headache attributable to the drug occurs in 8% (i.e. 10% minus 2%) of patients using it. In such trials it is also common to ask investigators whether or not they believe that individual events are related to the drug. This is effectively another way of collecting suspected ADRs, although such data are likely to be more complete if the patient is in a clinical trial rather than being treated in ordinary practice. It is important to realise that this remains a methodologically weaker approach. Providing that the estimated 8% difference was not based on very small numbers, then it would be much more persuasive evidence that the drug causes headache.

Thus, the three terms defined above should be applied in the following contexts:

- Use 'ADR' to mean that it is now generally accepted that drug x may cause effect y rather than in relation to individual cases. Qualify the term with 'possible' if there is doubt.
- Use 'suspected ADR' when a health professional or investigator indicates that a drug *may* have been responsible for an event in an individual case. A valid case submitted as a spontaneous report to a company or regulatory authority is a suspected ADR by definition.
- Use 'AE' only in the context of systematic data collection when no element of judgement is involved in determining whether or not a case is counted.

Classification systems

Since the 1970s, ADRs have traditionally been classified into two broad categories, as follows:
- Type A (Augmented) reactions
- Type B (Bizarre) reactions

The usual characteristics of these different types of reactions are contrasted below, followed by some examples.

Type A reactions are generally:
- Dose-related
- Predictable from drug pharmacology
- Common
- Normally reversible
- May be manageable with dose adjustment.

Classic examples of Type A reactions are bleeding with warfarin, hypoglycaemia with sulphonylureas and headache with glyceryl-trinitrate.

Type B reactions are generally:
- Not dose-related
- Unpredictable
- Uncommon
- May be serious/irreversible
- Indicative that the drug needs to be stopped.

Classic examples of Type B reactions are anaphylaxis with penicillins, hepatitis with halothane and agranulocytosis with clozapine.

Additional categories of ADRs have also been suggested, as follows:
- Type C (Chronic) – e.g. adrenal suppression with corticosteroids
- Type D (Delayed) – e.g. tardive dyskinesia with neuroleptics
- Type E (End of use) – e.g. withdrawal reactions with benzodiazepines

In 2003, a system of classification was proposed by Aronson and Ferner based on **dose-relatedness, time course** and **susceptibility;** this is known as 'DoTS'. The main ways in which ADRs may be classified within each of these three categories is given below:

Summary of DoTS categories

Dose	Time	Susceptibility
Toxic	Independent	Age
Collateral	Dependent	Gender
Hypersusceptibility	– rapid administration	Ethnic origin
	– first dose	Genetic
	– early, intermediate, late	Disease
	– delayed	
	– withdrawal	

In terms of dose-relatedness, 'toxic' means that reactions occur as a result of drug levels being too high, 'collateral' means that reactions occur at drug levels which are in the usual therapeutic range and 'hypersusceptibility' means that reactions may occur even at very low, sub-therapeutic doses. The terms early, intermediate and late have not been precisely defined; the main difference between 'late' and 'delayed' reactions is that the latter may occur long after treatment is stopped (e.g. cancer, which may occur years after exposure to a causal agent). A withdrawal reaction means one that is specifically precipitated by stopping the drug.

If suitable estimates of risk are available, it may be possible to draw three-dimensional DoTS diagrams of the probability of an ADR occurring in sub-groups over time and as a function of dose. When this is not possible, qualitative classification may still be useful, as shown by the following examples:

DoTS classification: examples

1 Osteoporosis due to corticosteroids:
This reaction occurs at therapeutic doses, usually after some months of treatment; females and older people are at the greatest risk. Hence it would be classified as:

Dose: collateral effect
Time: late
Susceptibility: age, sex
2 Anaphylaxis due to penicillin:
This reaction may occur with very small doses and within min-
utes of taking the first dose of a course, but true anaphylaxis only
occurs when the drug (or a closely related agent) has been used
previously. Hence it would be classified as:
Dose: hypersusceptibility
Time: first dose
Susceptibility: requires previous sensitisation
The DoTS approach seems to be gaining acceptance because
it addresses the limitations of the A/B scheme into which many
ADRs do not clearly fit. Furthermore, it is useful in providing
pointers as to how specific ADRs may be avoided.

Nature and mechanisms of ADRs
The adverse effects of medicines usually mimic diseases or
syndromes which occur naturally and have a variety of non-drug
potential causes, e.g. hepatitis or aplastic anaemia. However, there
are a few unique syndromes that, as far as we yet know, seem to
be caused only by specific drugs. Four examples of this are:
1 Vaginal cancer in teenagers caused by maternal exposure to stil-
  boestrol
2 Oculomucocutaneous syndrome caused by practolol
3 Eosinophilia-myalgia syndrome caused by some L-tryptophan
  products
4 Fibrosing colonopathy induced by large doses of high-strength
  pancreatic enzymes in children with cystic fibrosis.
As a general rule, therefore, considering other potential causes is
an important part of the assessment of a potential adverse effect.
  There are at least four broad mechanisms for ADRs:
1 Exaggerated therapeutic response at the target site (e.g. bleeding
  with warfarin)
2 Desired pharmacological effect at another site (e.g. headache
  with glyceryltrinitrate)
3 Additional (secondary) pharmacological actions (e.g. prolonga-
  tion of the QT interval on the electrocardiogram – many drugs)
4 Triggering an immunological response (e.g. anaphylaxis due to
  many drugs).

Particularly at the time they are first identified, the mechanism of many ADRs is unknown or incompletely understood. Some have a pharmacokinetic basis, e.g. impaired hepatic metabolism due to a genetic polymorphism or the effect of another medication taken concurrently, leading to increased plasma concentrations. Understanding genetic pre-dispositions is likely to be an important factor in determining how we might prevent ADRs in the future (see Chapter 8).

Predisposing factors for ADRs

The main clinical factors which increase the chance that patients will experience an adverse reaction are listed below:

- *Age* – the elderly and neonates are at greatest risk.
- *Gender* – women are generally at greater risk.
- *Ethnic origin* – may affect drug metabolism.
- *Impaired excretory mechanisms* – reduced hepatic and/or renal function.
- *Specific diseases* – e.g. asthma and beta-blockers[*].
- *Polypharmacy* – i.e. use of multiple drugs simultaneously, increasing the potential for drug interactions (see below).
- *Any previous history of an ADR.*

Drug interactions occur when the presence of one drug affects the activity of another. This may occur either because both drugs act through the same pathway(s) – these are called 'pharmacodynamic' interactions – or through effects on absorption, distribution, metabolism or excretion – 'pharmacokinetic' interactions. The result may be an adverse reaction or modified effectiveness. Some specific examples are given below:

- *Pharmacodynamic* – concomitant use of two drugs with similar effects [e.g. an angiotensin converting enzyme (ACE) inhibitor plus a 'potassium sparing' diuretic may result in hyperkalaemia and cardiac arrhythmias].
- *Absorption* – use of broad-spectrum antibiotics (e.g. penicillin) may, through an effect of bacterial flora in the gut, result in reduced absorption and effectiveness of oral contraceptives.
- *Distribution* – protein-bound drugs (e.g. phenytoin, aspirin) may displace each other resulting in an increased unbound (i.e. active) fraction of drug in plasma.

---

[*]This is a very important example since the effect of beta-blockers in patients with asthma is to constrict the airways and to counteract some of the treatments that the patient may be taking (e.g. beta-agonists). Giving a beta-blocker to an asthmatic patient can prove to be fatal.

- *Metabolism* – cimetidine, a drug which reduces gastric acid, inhibits the metabolism of warfarin and thereby increases its anticoagulant effect, leading to bleeding reactions.
- *Excretion* – amiodarone, an anti-arrhythmic drug, reduces excretion of, and therefore the dosage requirements for, digoxin – a drug widely prescribed to patients with cardiac disease.

Many drugs are metabolised by hepatic cytochrome P450 enzymes, the activity of which may be induced or inhibited by a wide variety of drugs. Their activity may also be affected by:

- *Herbal medicines* – e.g. St. John's Wort is an enzyme inducer and may reduce the effectiveness of various drugs including ciclosporin.
- *Dietary products* – e.g. grapefruit juice is an enzyme inhibitor and increases plasma concentrations of some calcium channel blockers, drugs which are used to treat hypertension and angina.

Public health burden and costs of ADRs

Despite the relative safety of modern medicines – compared to those used in the past – ADRs remain an important cause of morbidity and mortality. A study from the UK published in 2004 suggested that about 6.5% of hospital admissions are related to an ADR and estimated the annual cost to the National Health Service to be around £500 million. In 1998, a published study reported that ADRs are among the top six causes of death in the USA.

ADRs are certainly the most important form of iatrogenic (i.e. doctor-induced) disease. Many of the serious reactions that occur are well-recognised and potentially preventable – e.g. bleeding with warfarin, the upper gastrointestinal effects of NSAIDs. In public health terms, it is not newly introduced drugs that are responsible for most of the population burden of adverse drugs reactions but those whose safety profile is 'well-established' (see below).

The concept of safety

Definition

Safety may be defined as **relative absence of harm.** When using the word 'safety' we often mean something else. For example, 'safety' data often means collection of reports of harm. Safety departments in the pharmaceutical industry are generally focused much more on harm than safety. And yet how safe something is a key question for the user and one that pharmacovigilance is gradually becoming more targeted at. To establish safety, it is not enough to sit around and hope that nothing much happens. Active processes are required to generate data in large numbers of users – this is one of the main challenges facing people working in the field.

In practice, there is no such thing as absolute safety because, even if something is completely harmless, it is impossible to demonstrate that with complete certainty. For example, if a drug were given to 999,999 people without any problem occurring, it would be very unlikely that the millionth person to use it would be harmed, but it is not impossible. In any case, we know that all pharmacologically active substances have the potential to cause harm. When we say that a drug is 'safe', we mean that there is a low probability of harm that, *in the context of the disease being treated and the expected benefits of the drug*, can be considered acceptable. Disease context is important because patients with more serious illnesses are much more likely to be prepared to accept potentially harmful treatments than those who have minor or self-limiting illnesses. 'Acceptability' is a subjective judgement which ultimately is made by comparing both the positive and the negative consequences of one course of action (e.g. a drug) with another (which could be any form of treatment or no treatment). I will return to this point in more detail in the section on risk-benefit balance below.

Safety is a moving ball – there is a need to re-evaluate it as experience accumulates. Treatments previously considered acceptably safe may become 'unsafe' in the light of new evidence or the discovery of safer alternatives. An example of the latter was the antihistamine terfenadine which was widely used in the treatment of hay fever until the early 1990s. It was then discovered that it could, very rarely, cause serious or fatal ventricular arrhythmias through the mechanism of prolonging the QT interval on the electrocardiogram. Terfenadine is a 'pro-drug' which is normally completely metabolised on the 'first-pass' through the liver. It is the parent drug terfenadine that prolongs the QT interval (when its metabolism is inhibited) but the metabolite is responsible for the beneficial effects. Thus the metabolite, known as fexofenadine, was developed for this indication and rapidly accepted to be a safer alternative, following which terfenadine became obsolete.

To assess how safe something is we need to identify and measure the risks of harm associated with it. **Risk** is the probability of an adverse outcome. It may be expressed in the following terms:

- **Absolute risk** – An absolute risk must have a numerator and a denominator but it may be a proportion (e.g. 1 in 100) or a rate which includes time (e.g. 1 in 100 per year). The 'null value' is zero.
- **Relative risk** – A relative risk is a ratio and makes comparison with a specified alternative (e.g. a two-fold increase compared to no treatment is a relative risk of 2). The 'null value' is one.

Absolute risk is more useful information than relative risk but the latter is often easier to measure. Interpreting a relative risk is difficult without knowledge of the 'baseline' rate, i.e. the background probability of the effect occurring in the absence of any intervention. Several times a very small number is still a small number whereas a small increase in the relative risk of something common could be important. This is illustrated by the following comparison:

Baseline risk	Relative risk	No. of extra cases per million
1 in 100 (common)	1.1 (small increase)	1,000
1 in 1,000,000 (very rare)	10 (large increase)	10

The fundamental problem with safety is that it is much more difficult to determine that an effect is absent than to measure one that is present. We may be hoping or expecting to observe no effect but if nothing goes wrong, does that mean everything is alright? The **rule of three** is a simple and useful tool when zero cases have been observed in a defined population. Simply dividing the size of population by 3 approximates an upper 95% confidence limit. In practice, this is the highest value that, statistically, is reasonably likely to represent the truth. For example:

If 900 patients use a new antibiotic and 0 allergic reactions occur then it is statistically unlikely that such reactions will occur more frequently than 1 in 300 patients (i.e. 1 in 900/3).

The rule of three works very well provided the size of the population is at least 30 and thus, in the context of drug safety, it usually is applicable.

Safety in practice

There are two basic components to safety:
- **Intrinsic safety** – Some drugs are intrinsically and obviously safer than others at therapeutic doses. Compare, e.g., the adverse reactions produced by paracetamol and any cytotoxic drug.

- **User-dependent safety** – The safety of a drug usually depends on how it is used. For example, monitoring white blood cell count in users of clozapine can completely prevent progression of a reduction in white blood cells to a level that would potentially have fatal consequences. Using the drug without such monitoring is therefore clearly less safe than following the recommended procedure. Another example of safety being dependent on the user would be giving penicillin to someone who is allergic to it, perhaps because that information has been ignored or is not available. In such a case, the safeguard (i.e. means of minimising the risk) is avoidance of a specific drug in a particular individual. Using an appropriate dose of medicine is an example of practising risk minimisation that applies to most therapeutic situations.

The amount of safety knowledge available for a drug depends on how much it has been studied and used. Broadly, there are four categories of safety in respect of the amount of knowledge available, as follows:

1 **Well-established** – Drugs which have been widely used for many (~ 20+) years for which it is unlikely that *completely unidentified* safety issues will emerge.
2 **Established** – Drugs for which there is a substantial body of evidence of safety in clinical use but not enough to meet level 1 above.
3 **Provisional** – All newly authorised drugs until they have been used fairly extensively in ordinary practice over a period of at least two years. During this period such drugs should be monitored intensively and their safety in ordinary practice proactively studied.
4 **Limited** – All investigational drugs and the following situations where the drug might be authorised on limited safety information:
   - Small populations eligible for treatment – 'orphan drugs'.
   - Drugs with important benefits or where there is great clinical need, i.e. situations where potentially large risks might be acceptable.

A logical principle following from this categorisation is that *all* use of the drug should be associated with systematic collection of safety information.

It is important to recognise that drugs in the 'well-established category' are not necessarily safer than those in lower categories (and so on) – only that more information is available about their safety.

Risk-benefit balance

Since absolute safety is an unattainable goal, the aim is to use medicines with an **acceptable level of safety**. Various factors need to be considered in judging whether safety is or is not acceptable:

- The level of *absolute* risk(s) and the potential health consequences
- The benefit(s) expected, also measured in absolute terms
- The seriousness of the disease for which treatment is given
- The risks and benefits of alternative approaches
- The perspective of the individual who is to be exposed

In practice, therefore, whether or not safety is acceptable cannot be divorced from efficacy and expected benefits. The harms and benefits of a medicine are balanced at two levels:

1 The population level – this is a regulatory task and a question of whether, overall, the benefits that will accrue from availability of a medicine will exceed the expected harms.

2 The individual level – this is made by clinicians and patients and takes into account factors such as the patient's previous treatment, disease severity and preferences.

The process of balancing harms and benefits is a judgemental one and an element of judgement is always likely to remain, despite promising attempts that are currently being made to develop mathematical tools to aid the process at the population level. The term risk-benefit ratio has often been used but is best avoided. A ratio implies one number divided by another and even if two simple numbers were available to summarise risks and benefits, what would a ratio of, say, 1.5 mean? Conceptually it is preferable to use an additive process and the resulting balance becomes analogous to a financial balance which is either positive or negative. Ideally, a balance sheet would be constructed and the debits (i.e. the ADRs) would be subtracted from the credits (i.e. the expected benefits), hopefully leaving a positive balance. The problems are that the credits and debits are not usually measurable in the same way and there is often uncertainty about the size of some of the entries. Nevertheless, the analogy is conceptually helpful – i.e. to achieve these benefits it is reasonable (or not) to accept these risks of harm.

Causation – was the drug responsible?

Deciding whether or not a drug is responsible for an AE is very often the most important question facing scientists working in the field of pharmacovigilance. Yet, it is rarely completely straightforward whether the matter is being considered at the level of an individual patient or in terms of study data of various types. As in the case of the risk-benefit balance, a judgement is often necessary and there are some principles to be applied. There are some similarities in approach between the two levels mentioned above although they will be considered separately below.

Assessing causality in individual cases

Many causality algorithms and categorisation systems have been proposed but none has gained universal acceptance, and the value of assessing this for each individual report of a suspected ADR now seems to be doubtful. It is certainly much more efficient to reserve such assessment for a series of cases which might represent a new and/or important safety issue. Systematic assessment of causality in individual cases occurring in clinical trials is intrinsically a weaker approach to assessing causality than comparison of numerical counts.

When individual case causality assessment is to be performed, I would suggest using the following four categories into which a case might be placed:

- **Probable** – the balance of information available supports causation.
- **Possible** – some of the available information is in favour of and some against causation.
- **Unlikely** – the balance of information available is against causation.
- **Unassessable** – a reasonable judgement cannot be made, often because key information is missing.

In making such judgements there are four broad areas to consider:

- **Temporal relationships** – what was the time relationship between starting treatment and the onset of the event; if treatment was stopped ('dechallenge') or restarted ('rechallenge') did the event abate and/or recur?
- **Alternative causes** – are there concomitant diseases and medications or non-drug exposures that could explain the event?
- **Nature of the event** – some clinical events are often caused by drugs and immediately suggest a relationship (e.g. certain types of skin reactions).
- **Plausibility** – is the reaction already recognised with this drug (or similar drugs) or can a mechanism be postulated based on the pharmacology of the drug?

In terms of temporal association, sometimes causation can be considered definitely excluded – ADRs cannot start before the drug is given (although drugs can worsen existing diseases). On the other hand, a positive rechallenge in the absence of alternative causes is generally considered to be strong evidence for causation. Whilst most ADRs start early on in treatment this is not invariably true, as reflected in the time course element of the DoTS classification discussed above.

Merely because an alternative cause can be identified does not mean that it was responsible. Such potential causes are often called 'confounding factors' and when they are present, cases are said to be 'confounded'. This is rather loose use of the word (see Chapter 3) and best avoided.

The issues of nature of the event and plausibility need to be considered with some caution – these factors may add to the arguments for causation but a clinical event that is not normally known to be drug-related or the absence of any information supporting plausibility is not strong evidence against it.

Assessing causality from study data

One of the main reasons why data from randomised controlled trials are considered to be the 'gold standard' is that, in principle, observed differences between randomised groups should be attributable to the different treatments (i.e. causal). Other explanations are still possible, e.g. differences could simply be due to chance or caused by various biases, particularly in relation to what is being measured. Problems with the randomisation may also occur – e.g. it may not have been done properly. Sometimes, as a result of bad luck, randomisation may not have worked to produce groups that were adequately balanced at baseline in terms of important factors which may predict the outcome of interest. Whilst all these alternative explanations need to be considered, when a difference that looks important is observed in a randomised trial, causation is the most likely explanation. If the trial has adequate statistical power (and the difference is significant), the groups were well-balanced at baseline and the measurements are objective or blinded, then no great element of judgement is required to accept that such a treatment difference is likely to be real.

For study data which are not randomised, assessing causation requires much more judgement and is often a source of debate. When such studies find a difference this is known as an 'association'.

In terms of chance, the issues are much the same as for randomised trials but there are many more types of biases that may be relevant. In the real world people tend to do things for a reason and patients who are given particular treatments may be selected according to factors which are relevant to the outcome of interest. Losses to follow-up are more likely than in trials and the reasons why people are 'lost' from studies may not be random.

Aside from the greater problem of bias, there is also the problem of 'confounding'. A confounder has a triangular relationship with an exposure (usually a drug) and outcome (AE of interest). When it is present, the risk of the outcome is affected and whether or not it is present also varies according to the exposure status. Age is a good example of a perennial confounder – in very simple terms, older people tend to use more drugs and have more adverse outcomes. Therefore there is a need to be sure that any observed association is not simply a consequence of that. A randomised study will, unless it is small, tend to balance the groups for age – or indeed any confounder – largely circumventing this problem. In principle, confounding can be dealt with – either in the study design (e.g. by matching patients or groups so that relevant factors are balanced) or, more commonly, in the analysis by statistical adjustment. However, to do so requires that all potential confounders are identified and adequately measured. Smoking is another common confounder and knowledge of smoking status in terms of (say) current, ex- or non-smoker is fairly crude given that there may be a close relationship between the precise amount smoked and the risk of the outcome. The possibility that confounding has not been fully addressed is called 'residual confounding' and this is often a possible alternative explanation to causation when the data come from non-randomised studies.

When chance, bias and confounding are considered unlikely, causation is possible but still cannot be assumed as an explanation for an association based on non-randomised data. Often there may be a series of studies or various types of data which bear on this question. In this context, nine criteria first described by Bradford–Hill in the 1960s are still used. These may be summarised as follows:

Strength – the stronger an association is, the less likely is to be explained by other factors.

Consistency – repeated observation of an association in different studies and under different conditions support causation.

Specificity – a few ADRs are completely unique syndromes (some examples were given above) and their specificity means that causation is hardly in doubt.

Temporality – exposures must precede outcomes in a consonant manner.

Biologic gradient – is there evidence of dose- or duration-related risk?

The final four criteria are: plausibility, coherence, supportive experimental evidence and analogy – these are related by a theme of whether or not the association fits with existing scientific knowledge and beliefs. If so then causation is more likely but newly identified associations may not fit – so absence of any or all of these criteria does not preclude an association being causal.

In general terms, the more criteria that are met, the more likely an association is to be causal. However there is no simple formula for adding up these criteria and coming to a definitive answer. Judgement is required and Bradford–Hill's criteria are merely a conceptual framework for making such judgement. It is worth noting that some of the criteria, e.g. temporality, dose-response, plausibility, are analogous to what was described above for the assessment of causality in individual cases.

Conclusion

This chapter has considered the most fundamental concepts in pharmacovigilance, namely what is an adverse effect of a medicine, how do we know that it really is an adverse effect and on what basis do we consider a treatment to be safe? The next step is to consider in more detail the various kinds of data that help us to answer such questions in relation to specific medicines and safety issues.

CHAPTER 3
Types and sources of data

Introduction

The safety of medicines is under evaluation throughout the drug development cycle. This process starts before humans are exposed, and continues during the clinical development and post-marketing phases. Broadly, the safety of a medicine is tested in four phases, each of which produces different types of data. These are as follows:

- Pre-clinical (animal) studies
- Healthy human volunteer studies (Phase I)
- Clinical trials (Phases II and III)
- Post-marketing surveillance (Phase IV)

Although there is a natural sequence defined by the above order, the phases are not entirely distinct. Sometimes, new pre-clinical studies are undertaken for authorised products and, as we saw in Chapter 1, clinical trials are increasingly becoming important post-marketing. Systematic reviews and meta-analysis are important tools for bringing together data from multiple studies. Although they have usually been applied in the assessment of efficacy, their use for safety purposes is increasing.

Pre-clinical studies

Pre-clinical studies are usually conducted in rodents (rabbit, mouse, rat) and dogs. They aim to establish dosage levels below which toxicity is not observed and to identify the organs adversely affected by higher doses. The most important potential effects studied are:

- Major organ toxicity
- Chronic toxicity

An Introduction to Pharmacovigilance. By Patrick Waller.
Published 2010 by Blackwell Publishing, ISBN: 978-1-4051-9471-6.

- Carcinogenicity
- Mutagenicity (i.e. able to induce genetic mutation)
- Teratogenicity (i.e. producing physical defects in the embryo)

Even at this stage, some adverse effects might be acceptable depending on the ultimate target population for the drug. For example, adverse reproductive effects could be considered unimportant for a drug that is to be used exclusively in an elderly population.

ADRs may or may be not specific to particular species. When studies in animals demonstrate major toxicity, further drug development is usually precluded and the level of toxicity in humans remains unknown. When no major toxicity has been demonstrated in animals, development can proceed into man but some ADRs appear to be specific to humans (e.g. the multi-system oculomucocutaneous syndrome caused by the beta-blocker practolol).

Overall, the predictive value of pre-clinical studies for human toxicity is not more than moderate. Thus they provide only limited reassurance that use in humans will be acceptably safe.

Human volunteer studies

For most medicines, the first human exposure takes place in healthy volunteers (cytotoxic drugs used to treat cancers are an exception) and participants are very closely monitored with clinical supervision and resuscitation equipment immediately to hand. The purposes are to establish a possible dosage regimen, investigate how the drug is handled and what the effects are on a variety of standard parameters (e.g. pulse and blood pressure, ECG, haematology, etc.). Assuming the drug appears to have no major untoward effects, it can then be studied in clinical trials which include patients with the target disease(s).

Healthy volunteer (or Phase I) studies have generally had a good safety record over a long period of time but, occasionally, major adverse reactions do occur. In 2006, all six of the first humans treated with the monoclonal antibody TGN1412 at Northwick Park Hospital in London rapidly developed multi-organ failure. The incident was investigated in detail by the UK regulatory authority who concluded that the reactions were an unexpected biological effect.

Clinical trials

Clinical trials are usually designed to study both safety and efficacy. They incorporate various design features to minimise bias such as randomisation to treatment groups, blinding of subjects and observers to treatment allocation, and validated measurement instruments. Initially, fairly small studies known as Phase II trials are conducted – these tend to be focused on efficacy and dosage requirements. Larger, Phase III trials are then conducted and will form the key element of the safety database prior to marketing. All adverse events occurring in patients after exposure to the drug and a comparator (which may be a placebo or an alternative active drug) are systematically recorded. In order to minimise measurement bias it is usual to 'blind' all study participants (i.e. patients and clinicians) to the treatments given or, if that is not possible, to 'blind' those who are involved in assessing the outcomes, particularly if there is any subjectivity involved.

In clinical trials, the data are analysed to identify adverse events that occur at significantly higher rates on the drug of the interest than on comparators. Usually the data from all trials are pooled in a global safety analysis. Clinical trials will identify most common adverse reactions but often have important limitations, including:

• The numbers of patients studied is generally not enough to identify rare but serious ADRs.
• The duration of follow-up is usually short, i.e. weeks or months rather than years.
• Selection of patients – those at greatest risk of ADRs are often excluded.
• The artificial conditions – patients are likely to be more closely monitored than in real life.
• Measurement of surrogate markers of effect rather than 'hard' end-points.

At the conclusion of a clinical trial, patients may be continued on treatment and followed-up for a period of months or years, generating more long-term safety experience (these are known as open-label extensions). When clinical trials are conducted entirely after marketing, they may provide important new safety information provided that they contain enough patients, and have few exclusion criteria and clinically relevant outcomes that are easily measured (e.g. mortality). Such studies are often called 'large simple trials'.

During the clinical trial phase of development, there is a major safety focus on the protection of trial subjects. Investigators are obliged to document and report serious adverse events promptly. If serious, unexpected and suspected to be related to the drug (this is known as a 'SUSAR' – see Chapter 5), then a case should be unblinded and reported to regulatory authorities. The identification of a serious new hazard may lead to a trial or even the whole development programme being stopped. In many large trials there is a safety monitoring committee appointed to oversee unblinded safety results as they emerge, possibly in accordance with a pre-planned series of 'sequential' analyses. Care needs to be taken so that such procedures do not compromise the integrity of the trial, but the need to ensure that trial subjects are not exposed to unnecessary risk is paramount. In this respect there is an ethical dimension to safety in trials which will be considered further in Chapter 7.

Post-marketing surveillance

Because of the limitations of pre-marketing studies described above, safety can only be regarded as provisional when a new medicine is first marketed and there is a need to collect more evidence arising from 'real world' usage. Spontaneous ADR reporting is generally regarded as the cornerstone of such monitoring and its main purpose is for the detection of 'signals' of previously unrecognised hazards, i.e. hypothesis generation. Formal pharmacoepidemiological studies are then used to investigate and characterise serious possible ADRs, i.e. hypothesis testing. The extent to which the safety of a new drug can be studied post-marketing depends considerably on how much it is used. If uptake is slow then it may be some time before there is sufficient exposure to conduct a formal study. On the other hand, if uptake is rapid then many people may suffer the consequences of an important safety problem whilst it is being identified and investigated.

Spontaneous ADR reporting systems

The primary purpose of spontaneous ADR reporting is to provide early warnings or 'signals' of previously unrecognised drug toxicity. As discussed in Chapter 1, the method was developed in the 1960s in response to the thalidomide tragedy and is now well-established throughout the developed world and in some developing countries. Health professionals are the key original source of reports, but patient reporting is becoming more widely accepted although its value is yet unclear (see below). Electronic transmission of all reports is likely to become the norm within the next few years. This is well-advanced between pharmaceutical companies and regulatory authorities but much less so in terms of initial transmission from health professionals in many parts of the world.

Spontaneous ADR reporting may be defined as a scheme for collating individual case reports of clinical suspicions of ADRs operated for the primary purpose of detecting unknown, potentially seriously harmful effects of drugs. As discussed in Chapter 2, individual cases can be assessed for causation using established principles. However, except in the very rare circumstance whereby a drug causes a previously unidentified syndrome (i.e. an apparently completely specific drug-event association), a series of spontaneous ADR reports provides only limited evidence of causation. Generally therefore, data from these schemes raise questions rather than provide answers.

Extensive spontaneous ADR reporting systems are in operation around the world and these are generally effective but they are not a panacea for two main reasons. Firstly, the output is essentially only a 'signal', which is a possible association requiring further evaluation and investigation; some signals will inevitably turn out to be false positives, i.e. not related to the drug. Secondly, the method is far from perfect in rapidly detecting all unrecognised ADRs – i.e. there will also be false negatives which are ultimately detected by other methods (e.g. practolol and oculomucocutaneous syndrome, as discussed in Chapter 1).

Spontaneous ADR reporting is conceptually simple. Reports are submitted on a voluntary basis and information from them is entered onto a database which is screened regularly for signals. The main elements of a scheme which are essential to its success may be summarised as follows:

1 Health professionals who are willing to participate

The value of a spontaneous report mainly derives from the suspicion of a clinician that a drug may have been responsible for a particular event. Thus, when a report is derived from a patient or carer, it should be followed-up via the clinician. Co-operation from clinicians is therefore essential and, in practice, reporting is invariably voluntary. Although some countries theoretically have 'mandatory' ADR reporting schemes for health professionals, they do not have markedly higher reporting rates per head of the population, presumably because no practical mechanism of enforcement has yet been developed. The reasons why some health professionals are prepared to report seems to be altruistic and there is general agreement that paying them to report would be a step in the wrong direction.

2 Simplicity in submission of reports

If busy health professionals are to submit reports voluntarily, they are only likely to do so if the process is straightforward. Reporting needs to be facilitated by the ready availability of clearly laid out forms which are simple to complete, and internationally agreed standard forms are in wide use. Both paper and electronic forms need to be made available, the former with free postage. Some reports start with a telephone enquiry but follow-up to obtain written documentation is essential.

3 Prompt entry of reports onto a database

Unless a scheme receives very few reports, entry onto a computer database is vital and signals are unlikely to be detected until the relevant reports have been entered. It is, therefore, important to ensure prompt data entry and to avoid backlogs that could potentially contain vital new information. Standard dictionaries should be used for coding, in particular Medical Dictionary for Drug Regulatory Affairs (MedDRA) which is now the international standard medical terminology. A drugs dictionary is also required and the most commonly used is the one maintained by the World Health Organisation which uses the anatomical-therapeutic-chemical (ATC) classification system and contains around 50,000 drugs.

4 Follow-up of serious reports

Reporters may be contacted for 'follow-up' – i.e. provision of additional detailed clinical information (e.g. results of investigations, autopsy reports, etc.) or ascertainment of the outcome subsequent to initial submission. In most schemes follow-up is selective, dependent on the perceived importance of a report and the extent to which information important for its evaluation has already been provided. A simple principle is that all serious reports should be followed-up.

5 Analytical tools to detect signals

In the past decade there have been major advances in the application of analytical methods to detect to signals from spontaneously reported ADRs (see Chapter 4). The general view is that these tools are now sufficiently well-established to be regarded as an essential component of the method but there are some sceptics.

6 Processes for dealing with signals

Once a signal has been identified, the next step is to evaluate all the relevant available information, including that derived from other data sources. Because signal evaluation is resource-intensive and large numbers of signals may be detected in some databases, interim steps have been proposed to prioritise them including 'triage' and impact analysis. These tools and the principles of signal evaluation are discussed in Chapter 4.

7 Feedback to reporters

In order to complete a feedback loop, information must also flow back to reporters through acknowledgement, provision of data and bulletins describing evaluated signals.

Spontaneous reporting schemes are well-established throughout the developed world and have also been set up in some developing countries. Most national schemes are run by the medicines regulatory agency but other models exist, e.g. in the Netherlands where the monitoring centre is a separate institution. Some larger countries have regional centres which may serve as a local base for the submission, handling and follow-up of reports, and/or assist in promoting reporting and education about ADRs. In France, the whole country is covered by such regional centres with a relatively small co-ordinating group based at the French medicines agency. In the UK, only part of the country is covered by regional centres.

In most countries pharmaceutical companies have legal obligations to submit spontaneous adverse reaction reports (see Chapter 5) and these are entered onto the national database. There is some variation between countries as to the proportion of reports which come via the industry (e.g. a large majority do so in Germany and the USA but the proportion is less in the UK). There is a potential for duplication of reports which a clinician submits to both industry and agency and also because more than one clinician may report the same case. A systematic approach to screening databases for duplicates is required and this task has become more difficult in recent years as confidentiality restrictions have increased.

International standards for ADR reporting have been developed since the late 1980s through the Council for the International Organisation of Medical Sciences (CIOMS) and International Conference on Harmonisation (ICH) – see Chapter 6.

The main strengths of spontaneous reporting lie in its simplicity, that it can be universally applied (all drugs, all the time) and in its ability to rapidly capture clinical suspicions that may otherwise to go unrecorded. In theory, spontaneous reporting is cheap to run although, globally, a lot of resource is now put into it and, overall, it is not as efficient as it could be because of duplicated efforts.

The main limitations of the method revolve around inevitable and unquantifiable under-reporting, and the potential for the data to be misunderstood. Curiously, most of the biases affecting the data are actually positive features which reflect the way these schemes are promoted. Thus a report is more likely to be submitted if the ADR is serious, unrecognised or relates to a new drug – all features which are desirable. The other major bias – the effect of publicity – is generally undesirable but can only occur once a hazard has been recognised by some means. It therefore does not detract from the primary purpose of the method but it does mean that interpretation of the data during subsequent monitoring is fraught with difficulty. Misperceptions of the data are common – e.g. the information that (say) 50 fatal suspected ADRs have been reported with a particular drug sounds worrying, particularly to lay people. However, this cannot be interpreted without considering carefully several factors, including the nature of the possible ADRs, what the drug is used for, how much it has been used and what other evidence might be available to support a causal link. Spontaneous ADR databases contain a fair amount of background 'noise', i.e. suspected reactions that were not actually caused by the drug but this point is often not appreciated by lay people.

It is important to recognise that spontaneous ADR reporting is most likely to detect signals of relatively rare ADRs when the background incidence of the disease is low. Relatively common ADRs are likely to have been detected earlier in drug development by clinical trials and detecting rare ADRs is difficult when the background incidence of the event is high. This is because clinicians are not surprised to see cases of common diseases.

Although spontaneous ADR reporting is a well-established method, both the utility of the schemes and the data they generate are frequently subject to misperceptions. For example, a report prepared by politicians in 2005 described the UK scheme as 'widely considered to be failing', an assessment which no scientist experienced in the field would accept. One of the main reasons for this assessment seems to be the problem of under-reporting but this is inherent in the method. There seem to be some widely held myths about under-reporting which can be questioned. The first is that the overall degree of under-reporting approximates to 90%, i.e. 10% of ADRs are reported. The evidence base for this is very limited and the reality is that the degree of under-reporting varies considerably in relation to factors such as seriousness, the novelty of the drug and the nature of the suspected ADR. Critics also seem to believe that the effectiveness of these schemes might be directly proportional to the number of reports received and even that under-reporting undermines the whole concept. These perceptions are not based on hard evidence and do not reflect around

45 years of experience with the method. The main solution proposed by critics of spontaneous reporting schemes is patient reporting. The argument is that if health professionals would not report then patients should be allowed to do so.

To date, there have been relatively few studies of patient reporting and it is not possible to be sure of its value. It will not be sufficient just to show that numbers of reports can be increased (there is little reason to doubt that) but also that the data are useful, i.e. signals of important toxicity can be detected earlier than in the absence of patient reports. There are two major potential downsides to patient reporting – firstly the extra resources involved, secondly the potential for losing support from health professionals who may feel undermined. This has become a political rather than a scientific issue and it would be ironic if well-meaning attempts to improve the method turned out to make it less effective.

Despite the limitations discussed, it is clear that we will continue to need systems that fulfil the purpose of spontaneous ADR reporting schemes for the foreseeable future. It is also clear that, for most drugs, relying on spontaneous reporting alone is insufficient and a proactive approach to studying safety using pharmacoepidemiological studies is needed.

Pharmacoepidemiological studies

Pharmacoepidemiology is the scientific discipline of studying drug effects in populations which is largely focused on measuring potential harms and safety in the post-marketing phase. Pharmacoepidemiological studies are 'observational' (whereas clinical trials are 'experimental' or 'interventional') – they attempt to measure effects under real-life conditions. Larger populations can be studied than in clinical trials and the findings are likely to be generally applicable. However, as discussed in Chapter 2, without randomisation, attribution of causation is more difficult. Observational studies provide evidence of association (or no association) and a judgement then has to be made on causation taking into account all the available information. To recap from Chapter 2, four possible explanations for a positive association generally have to be considered:

- Chance (taking into account the level of statistical significance)
- Bias (a systematic error)
- Confounding (the association is produced by a third factor which is related to both drug use and outcome)

- Causal effect (the other explanations can reasonably be excluded, as assessed by Bradford–Hill's criteria when the other explanations can reasonably be excluded)

The two principal types of study design used are as follows:

- **Cohort study** – all users of a drug are identified and followed-up to determine what events or ADRs occur.
- **Case–control study** – all cases of the disease, i.e. the putative reaction, are identified and their use of the drugs of interest is compared to controls without this disease.

A case-control study may be 'nested' within a cohort study, i.e. cases and controls are all drawn from a clearly defined cohort. This is an efficient design which is now commonly used in pharmacoepidemiology. Attempts are made in the design and analysis to minimise possible biases, and to identify and adjust for confounding factors. Typically a cohort study will measure both absolute and relative risks whereas a case-control study will usually only measure odds ratios which generally approximate to relative risks. In both cases the data may be summarised in two-by-two tables, as shown in the following examples:

Example of risk data from a cohort study design

	Used drug	No drug	Totals
Event	50 (a)	20 (b)	70
No event	9,950 (c)	9,980 (d)	19,930
Totals	10,000 (a + c)	10,000 (b + d)	20,000

Risk of event on drug: $a/(a + c)$ or $50/10,000 = 0.5\%$

Risk of event in comparison group: $b/(b + d)$ or $20/10,000 = 0.2\%$

Absolute risk attributable to drug: $[a/(a + c)] - [b/(b + d)]$ or 0.5% minus $0.2\% = 0.3\%$

Relative risk: $[a/(a + c)]/[b/(b + d)]$ or $0.5\%/0.2\% = 2.5$

Note that the starting point is two cohorts of 10,000 subjects who are followed-up and that relatively few of them (as is usually the case) experience the outcome of interest. The key estimate from this study is the attributable risk of 0.3% which means that about 1 patient in 333 (i.e. the inverse of 0.3%) will experience the event because of the drug, if the association is causal. The relative risk of 2.5 merely means that two and half times as many drug-treated patients experienced the event in comparison with those who did not receive the drug.

Example of risk data from a case-control study design

	Cases	Controls	Totals
Used drug	10 (a)	20 (b)	30
No drug	90 (c)	480 (d)	570
Totals	100	500	600

Odds ratio (approximate relative risk) = ad/bc = 4800/1800 = 2.67

Note that the starting point here is a series of identified cases of the outcome of interest. Prior exposure to the drug is then evaluated but only a few of the cases had used the drug. It is usual to include more controls since they are easier to find. Proportionately fewer controls had used the drug and therefore the odds ratio in this study was more than two. Since the odds ratio approximates to a relative risk, these two studies give a similar answer but, as discussed in Chapter 2, the additional information provided by the cohort study that the absolute risk is 0.3% is very useful.

Pharmacoepidemiological studies can be set up from scratch (so-called 'field' studies) but they are now normally conducted by using data collected for other purposes, e.g. from the General Practice Research Database in the UK or various health maintenance organisations in the USA.

In order to be useful for pharmacoepidemiological purposes a database must provide:
• Prescription records
• Event data
• Demographic and other health information
Studies can be done solely using information on a database, particularly if the quality of the data has been validated. However, it is often considered good practice to seek additional information from clinical records particularly to confirm that there is adequate evidence to support the diagnosis in individual cases. This may lead to some potential cases being excluded and exclusions may be specified for other reasons but, in general, these should be kept to a minimum in order to retain the advantage that such data have in representing real life.

Prescription event monitoring (PEM) is a pharmacoepidemiological system which uses the cohort design and was developed in England around 1980. It is mostly focused on new medicines, particularly those used for chronic diseases and is complementary to spontaneous reporting as a method of identifying unexpected ADRs.

PEM has the advantage that the number of users is known and therefore that event frequencies can be quantitated. An important point about the method is that all *events* are recorded, whether or not there is suspicion that they were drug-induced. PEM may therefore identify effects that clinicians do not recognise as being ADRs. It can also be used to investigate potential safety issues which have been identified during development.

In PEM, patients taking specific medicines are identified through prescriptions written by general practitioners (GPs). Events which occur during the subsequent 6–12 months are then captured on 'green forms' which are sent to and completed by GPs. The scheme is operated by the Drug Safety Research Unit (an independent charitable trust) and, to date, around 100 drugs have been studied by this method. The usual size of the cohort in PEM is about 10,000 patients – almost an order of magnitude greater than the usual number studied in clinical trials. When a medicine has been studied by PEM and no important new ADRs have been identified, the data provide some reassurance about its safety. However, PEM studies are not large enough to identify very rare ADRs. Like spontaneous reporting the PEM scheme is voluntary and it has received excellent co-operation from GPs. PEM has also proved to be feasible and valuable in Japan and New Zealand.

Registries

A registry is used to collect individual patient data which can be used for epidemiological studies. Ideally, it will provide complete capture of a sub-population based on a disease, treatment or outcome. Registries are particularly useful for studying long-term effects, rare diseases and rare exposures. With regard to drug safety, some examples of registries are as follows:

Disease/outcome based

- Cancer
- Orphan diseases

Drug-based

- As part of a risk minimisation programme (e.g. clozapine monitoring scheme)
- Drugs used to treat orphan diseases
- Patients who become pregnant whilst using a drug and the outcomes

A registry which has been used to collect data on biological therapies for rheumatoid arthritis is an example of one which is based on both disease and drugs. Registries which are disease-based offer greater flexibility in terms of study design – patients not exposed to particular drugs are useful for comparative purposes.

Systematic reviews and meta-analysis

These are increasingly important tools in 'evidence-based' medicine and their underlying purpose is to guide health and treatment policies, and the future research agenda.

A systematic review brings together and evaluates all the relevant research relating to a particular question. A group known as the 'Cochrane Collaboration' has been formed for the purpose of appraising medical treatments and publish its finding in the Cochrane Library which is available, freely in some countries, on the internet. Most of the focus has so far been on evidence of efficacy from randomised trials but an adverse event methods group has recently been formed.

A meta-analysis brings together data from different studies in a quantitative way so as to provide a single overall estimate of a specified effect. When doing this, it is best to use only evidence of one particular type (e.g. from randomised trials) and the outcome(s) must be expressed in the same terms for all the studies. Whilst meta-analysis has also been most often focused on efficacy, it can be used for adverse outcomes and the method is increasingly contributing to drug safety issues. Meta-analysis of data from observational studies is possible but more controversial than for randomised controlled trials.

A meta-analysis is, in effect, a 'study of studies' and it should be conducted according to a defined protocol. As far as possible, all the relevant evidence should be included whether published or not but duplication has to be avoided. In the presentation of data, the individual study findings ought to be demonstrated in addition to the overall effect. Meta-analysis is not the same as simple pooling of data from several studies. Rather than merely pooling the numerators and denominators, a meta-analysis combines the observed *differences* between treatments for each study and weighs them according to the precision of the studies so that the larger studies carry more weight.

As well as providing a combined estimate, a meta-analysis should aid understanding of the strengths and limitations of the available evidence. It is important to consider the reasons why the individual studies appear to differ in their findings. If there is a large degree of 'heterogeneity' in the data it is still possible to display that graphically but it may not be sensible to calculate a single overall estimate.

Conclusion

This chapter has considered the main types of data which are used in pharmacovigilance and their strengths and limitations. In the next chapter, I shall try to illustrate how such data fit into the overall process.

CHAPTER 4

The process of pharmacovigilance

Overview – a risk management process

As indicated in Chapter 1, pharmacovigilance is essentially a risk management process for medicines. The process starts with identification of a possible hazard, this is then evaluated and investigated and, if necessary, some action is then taken with a view to minimising risk. Implementation requires tools for communicating with users and the final step should be that an assessment of effectiveness is made. The process is iterative because new evidence may emerge or the measures taken may turn out to be insufficient. Rarely can a drug safety issue be considered completely and permanently resolved.

As already indicated, the start of the process is usually a 'signal', i.e. something that needs to be looked at further and which may or may not turn out to be a true hazard. Before that can happen, there is a need to identify the signal.

Signal detection

What is a signal?

The WHO has defined a signal as 'Reported information on a possible causal relationship between an adverse event and a drug, the relationship being unknown or incompletely documented previously. Usually more than a single report is required to generate a signal, depending upon the seriousness of the event and the quality of the information'. This definition seems entirely focused on spontaneous ADR reporting data and a broader approach would be to consider a signal as simply an alert from any available data

An Introduction to Pharmacovigilance. By Patrick Waller.
Published 2010 by Blackwell Publishing, ISBN: 978-1-4051-9471-6.

source that a drug *may* be associated with a previously unrecognised hazard or that a known hazard *may* be quantitatively (e.g. more frequent) or qualitatively (e.g. more serious) different from existing knowledge.

In practice, most signals will relate to previously unrecognised hazards, but a striking example of a signal that a known hazard was more serious than previously thought occurred in the mid-1990s. The non-steroidal anti-inflammatory drug, tiaprofenic acid, had been known to cause cystitis for over a decade but a series of cases was then reported indicating that, if the reaction was not recognised and the drug was continued in the long term, severe chronic cystitis might occur. The outcome was that surgical resection of the bladder was often necessary, leading to permanent disability.

Whilst some signals may be detected passively (e.g. from the medical literature), the process of signal detection should be fundamentally an active one. In terms of finding signals in large databases, it has been suggested that this is akin to looking for a needle in a haystack although there are likely to be lots of needles to find. The term 'data mining' is now widely used in this context, particularly in relation to systematic detection of signals from large spontaneous ADR databases.

Processes for signal detection

In the context of spontaneous ADR reporting, a signal is normally a series of cases of similar suspected ADRs reported in relation to a particular drug. When the suspected ADR is a disease which is rare in the general population (e.g. aplastic anaemia, toxic epidermal necrolysis), a very small number of cases associated with a single drug is unlikely to be a chance phenomenon, even if the drug has been used quite widely. Except for certain types of event that are particularly important and likely to be drug related (e.g. anaphylaxis), a single case is not usually sufficient to raise a signal. Three cases are generally considered to be the minimum number of cases needed.

The amount of drug usage (i.e. some drug exposure data) is helpful in providing some context to a series of reported cases but it is not usually critical in determining whether or not there is a signal which needs to be evaluated. The strength of evidence for the individual cases will be important to consider later but, initially, the key issue is whether or not there is an unexpectedly large enough number of cases.

In the past, various methods have been used to detect signals using spontaneous reporting data. Calculating reporting rates based on usage denominator data, either as prescriptions dispensed or defined daily doses, may enable a signal of a particular ADR to be derived by comparison with alternative treatments. Since spontaneous ADR reporting schemes are subject to a variable and unknown degree of under-reporting, such comparisons are crude. They may also be biased, particularly if the drugs being compared have been marketed for different indications or durations, or if there has been significant publicity about the adverse effects of one of the drugs.

The other principal approach that has been for making comparisons between drugs is to use the proportions of all ADRs for a particular drug that are of a specific type – perhaps within an organ system class of reactions (e.g. gastrointestinal or cutaneous). This is known as 'profiling', a method that has an advantage over reporting rates in that it is independent of the level of usage. The data may be displayed graphically as 'ADR profiles'. This proportionate approach forms the basis of statistical methods which have been developed since the mid-1990s and are now widely used. One important advantage of these methods is that no external data (e.g. usage) are required – they are entirely based on information present on a single database.

The basic concept behind such measures of 'disproportionality' is whether or not more reports have been received for a particular drug-reaction combination that might have been expected as background noise. When all drugs are considered together, large ADR databases tend to have fairly stable proportions of particular reactions over time. That proportion is used as a baseline for comparison – that is to determine what would be expected if there was no signal. In the UK Yellow Card database in mid-1990s, there were nearly 600,000 suspected reactions which had been reported to any drug over a period of 30 years. Almost 800 of these were classified as 'uveitis' – about 0.13%. A few years earlier, a new anti-tuberculous drug rifabutin had been introduced and some 41 cases of uveitis were reported as suspected ADRs to this drug. In total, only 55 reactions of any kind had been reported with rifabutin by that time (i.e. 75% of them were uveitis). In this example our expected proportion (derived from lumping all other drugs together) was therefore 0.13% but the observed value was 75%. Dividing 75/0.13 yields a number well over 500 – this is known as 'the proportional reporting ratio' (PRR). The 'null value' of a PRR is 1 and the calculation is made from a 2×2 table, as shown below:

Example of PRR calculation: rifabutin and uveitis

	Rifabutin	All Other Drugs	Totals
Uveitis	41	754	795
All other ADRs	14	591,958	591,972
Totals	55	592,712	592,767

Proportion of ADRs which are uveitis with rifabutin = 41/55 (i.e. 0.75).
Proportion of ADRs which are uveitis for all drugs 754/592,712 = 0.0013.
PRR = 0.75/0.0013 = 556.
Chi-squared (1 degree of freedom) = 22,000, $P \ll 0.00001$.

As can be seen from the statistical tests, this was very unlikely to have occurred by chance and is a very extreme finding. In fact, this signal was quite obvious without using any mathematics. The approach is more likely to be useful in identifying signals that might otherwise be missed when the PRR is much lower – say in the range 1–10. In general, experience has shown that a PRR of 3 or more represents a degree of disproportionality worth looking into further, providing it is unlikely to have occurred by chance, i.e. the value of chi-squared exceeds 4 (roughly the 5% level of statistical significance). Harking back to the point made above about generally needing three cases, it is therefore possible to regard the following as cut-off points for a minimum signal:

- PRR > 3
- Chi-squared > 4
- $N = 3$ or more

Using such criteria whole databases can be screened regularly by calculating 2×2 tables for all drug-reaction combinations to identify those that most need further attention.

A useful way of visualising the data is to plot, on logarithmic scales, the PRR against the value of chi-squared using the number of reports (N) as the symbol (Figure 4.1). The vertical and horizontal lines represent the cut-off points and everything in the upper right-hand quadrant is a signal of an unexpected degree of disproportionality. Note that the 41 cases of uveitis reported with rifabutin appear in this quadrant as one of the most extreme data points.

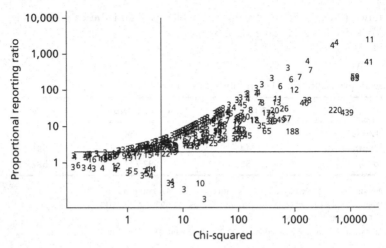

Figure 4.1 Plot of PRR vs. Chi-squared (from UK spontaneous ADR reporting data).

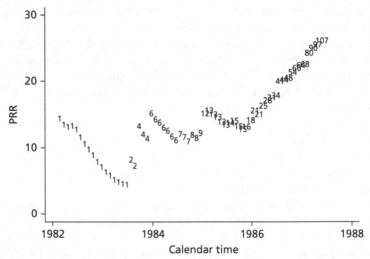

Figure 4.2 Plot of PRR over time for captopril and cough (from UK spontaneous ADR reporting data).

Another useful way of looking at the data is to plot the PRR over time (Figure 4.2). In this historical example, the ACE inhibitor captopril was first marketed in 1982 and it took until 1986 before cough was recognised as an adverse reaction with this class of drugs. Like thalidomide and practolol, the first indication of this association appeared in the literature. By the beginning of 1986 there were at least 15 reports in the UK and the criteria discussed above would have been met some 2 years earlier. Note how the PRR fluctuates over time – ADR databases are dynamic – and that the increase in the period 1986–1988 is an effect of publicity about the reaction.

The PRR is just one of several measures of disproportionality that have been used. A reporting odds ratio (ROR) can be calculated from the same 2×2 table and has been mostly used in the Netherlands. The WHO uses the Information Component (IC) and the US Food and Drugs Administration the Multi-Item Gamma Poisson Shrinker (MGPS), both of which are more complex measures based on Bayesian statistics. These measures tend to produce less extreme values than PRRs when the number of cases is very small. However, when the sensitivity, specificity and predictive power of these measures were compared using Dutch data in 2002, no important differences were found provided at least 3 cases had been reported.

A number of points about these methods are worth emphasising. First, although the numbers are calculated in a similar way to relative risks, they do not represent a meaningful calculation of risk. Whilst it is true that the greater the degree of disproportionality, the more reason there is to look further, the only real utility of the numbers is to decide whether or not there are more cases than might reasonably have been expected.

Indicators of disproportionality are measures of association and even quite extreme results may not be causal. The next step is clinical review of the relevant cases and to assess any other relevant information which may be available (see later). Many practitioners do not regard mathematical disproportionality alone as sufficient to raise a 'signal'. Thus, use of the terms 'statistical signal' and 'signal of disproportionate reporting' is emerging.

Aside from such semantic considerations, the underlying nature of the data and various potential biases inherent in spontaneous ADR reporting must not be forgotten. One specific problem arising from proportionate methods is that large effects may swamp and therefore mask smaller ones. It is fairly obvious that PRRs calculated for all the other suspected reactions reported with rifabutin (the example given earlier) are going to be less than 1 but it is quite possible that some of these reactions would also be worth looking into further.

The data mining approach to signal detection has been questioned in some quarters by practitioners who believe that relying on clinical experience alone is preferable but this seems to be an outlying view.

Evaluation and investigation

Signal prioritisation

Systematic use of data mining tools in a large spontaneous ADR database will identify large numbers of statistical signals. Evaluating all of them in detail would have major resource implications but many will turn out not to be real or to require no action. Possible signals have often been evaluated or dismissed on the basis of subjective judgements but two methods of prioritisation have been proposed:

1 **Triage** by the WHO
2 **Impact analysis** by the UK regulatory authority (MHRA)

Triage is analogous to a process used in emergency medicine to decide on priorities – essentially it is a quick look at the most important features of a case to decide on the urgency of further assessment and treatment relative to other cases. Impact analysis is more quantitative and involves calculating two scores which are then used to decide an overall priority. These are:

1 Evidence score
   • based on the degree of disproportionality (e.g. value of PRR)
   • strength of evidence
   • plausibility
2 Public health score
   • based on number of reported cases per year
   • expected health consequences
   • reporting rate in relation to level of drug exposure

The overall categories derived from these scores are as follows:
• **High priority** – prompt further evaluation is required
• **Need to gather more information**

- **Low priority**
- **No action**

It is important to recognise that these scores are only a means of deciding whether further evaluation is currently warranted and that impact analysis can and should be repeated if more evidence emerges.

Principles of signal evaluation

The data giving rise to the signal – whether arising from a series of individual cases or a formal study – should be evaluated in detail first. It is also important to consider what other immediately available data might be relevant, to obtain it and to include it in the evaluation. For example, are there any cases at all of the putative ADR (or similar clinical events) in randomised trials or are there any relevant pre-clinical findings? Are there any epidemiological data which might help or is there anything in the published literature?

When evaluating a signal the key issues are:

- Causality – assessed as discussed in Chapter 2, does the balance of evidence support cause and effect?
- Frequency – if this is a real effect, can we make any estimate of the likely level of absolute risk (usually in terms of an order of magnitude – see later)?
- Clinical implications (i.e. seriousness) – are there any fatal cases, is the reaction potentially life-threatening, can it result in long-term disability?
- Preventability – are there any factors which, even at this stage, suggest a potential means to prevent the adverse reaction or serious outcomes arising from it?

In terms of frequency, the following descriptors are generally used, based on orders of magnitude and expressed as a simple proportion of patients affected:

- **Very common** – more than 1 in 10
- **Common** – 1 in 10 to 1 in 100
- **Uncommon** – 1 in 100 to 1 in 1,000
- **Rare** – 1 in 1,000 to 1 in 10,000
- **Very rare** – less than 1 in 10,000

The outcome of signal evaluation is often that there is a need for further investigation, for example, of an epidemiological nature as described in Chapter 3. But there can also be enough evidence and concern to take action without waiting for confirmatory studies or, in some cases, it may not be feasible to conduct further studies, for example, because no suitable resource is available with data on enough patients.

Investigation

Primarily, signals are further investigated to provide more information about the key issues in signal evaluation – i.e. try to gain better evidence on whether the drug really does cause the effect, how common it is, how serious it is and how it might be prevented. In respect of the latter, this is often a question of trying to identify who is at particular risk of the adverse effect (i.e. what are the risk factors). Thus, as discussed in Chapter 3, pharmacoepidemiological studies are the main way in which signals are investigated.

The other common avenue of investigation is through mechanistic studies – through the application of basic science in the laboratory, can we understand the mechanism? Knowing, for example, that an adverse effect mostly occurs in people who are poor metabolisers of specific hepatic cytochrome substrates could be important in developing preventive measures.

Taking action

Potential options

The ultimate purpose of pharmacovigilance is prevention and therefore the actions which are taken will generally be intended to help prevent the occurrence of ADRs. There are many factors which may impact on the potential for prevention of ADRs. Broadly these may be classified into characteristics of the user or the drug. For example:

1 User characteristics
  - Demographics: age, sex, race
  - Genetic factors: polymorphisms (e.g. acetylator status)
  - Concomitant diseases (e.g. impaired hepatic or renal failure)
  - History of previous ADRs (e.g. allergy)
  - Compliance
2 Drug characteristics
  - Route of administration
  - Formulation (e.g. sustained vs. immediate release, excipients)

- Dosage regimen
- Therapeutic Index
- Mechanisms of drug metabolism and route of excretion
- Potential for drug interactions

Based on these possibilities, a wide variety of potential actions may be considered and in various combinations. It is useful to think of these in relation to the structure of the summary of product characteristics (SPC) – sections 4.1–4.9 and the potential amendments which might be made. For example:

Section of SPC	Examples
Indications/Uses	Limiting the indications to particular conditions with the greatest benefits by removal of indications (a) for which the benefits are insufficient to justify use (b) for which use is associated with a greater risk of the ADR
Dosing instructions	Reductions in dose (may be applied to specific groups e.g. the elderly); limitations on duration or frequency of treatment (especially for ADRs related to cumulative dose); provision of information on safer administration
Contra-indications	Addition of concomitant diseases and/or medications for which the risks of use are expected to outweigh the benefits
Warnings/ Precautions	Addition of concomitant diseases and/or medications for which the risks of use need to be weighed carefully against the benefits; additional or modified recommendations for monitoring patients
Interactions	Addition of concomitant medications or foods which may interact; advice on co-prescription and monitoring
Pregnancy/Lactation	Addition of new information relating to effects on the fetus or neonate; revised advice about use in these circumstances based on accumulating experience
Effects on driving	Practical advice on possible impairment of co-ordination
Undesirable effects	Addition of newly-recognised ADRs; improving information about the nature, frequency and severity of effects already listed
Overdosage	Adverse effects of overdosage; management, including the need for monitoring

Thus, it can be seen that every section of the clinical advice in the SPC might potentially need to be modified in relation to a new drug safety issue.

Apart from amending the advice to users, there are two more drastic types of action that might be considered. The first is to take some steps, beyond mere recommendation, to ensure that a key part of advice is, in practice, implemented. The second is to remove the drug from the market. A good example of the former is the scheme which was set up to ensure that users of the antipsychotic drug clozapine have their white blood cell counts effectively monitored. In essence, further supply of the drug was linked to the availability of a blood test result (i.e. no blood, no drug). The reason why this was done was that it had been demonstrated that regular blood tests would generally pick up a falling white blood cell count before patients developed serious infections and also that, on stopping the drug, the process was reversible.

Over a period of many years, about 4% of drugs put on the market have had to be withdrawn for safety reasons – a fairly low proportion. This reflects reluctance to use this draconian measure unless it is clear that, relative to alternative treatments, the risks outweigh its benefits despite maximum attempts to minimise the risks (and maximise the benefits). Withdrawal from the market is particularly problematic for drugs which are used chronically by large numbers of patients. If the adverse effect tends to occur early in treatment, established users will have a relatively low risk of the ADR – the main need is to prevent new starters. Existing regulatory systems do not readily address this dilemma although in some instances it is possible for patients using a withdrawn medicine to continue it on a 'compassionate use' basis.

When considering such decisions in the face of uncertain data it may be necessary to take into account the impact of the 'precautionary principle'. Whilst, scientifically, it may seem unsatisfactory to act decisively on unconfirmed risks – the need being for more data – some decisions may have to be made in advance of definitive data, and the precautionary principle is well-established in many areas of regulation. In particular, patients should not be expected to take a possible additional risk when there is no evidence of possible advantage in doing so. On the other hand, removing a drug from the market may mean that it becomes almost impossible to study it further and that clear answers will never be forthcoming. Thus, this is a 'Catch-22' situation but the main loser when a drug is withdrawn will be the manufacturer, unless the drug has particular benefits not shared by alternative treatments.

Making a decision

The first step in making a decision about how to manage an important drug safety issue is to bring together all the relevant evidence into a single document. This is usually called a risk-benefit report and there is an internationally agreed structure which has been defined in a report published by the CIOMS IV working group (see Chapter 6). Both companies and regulatory authorities use experts, often in the form of a Committee, to review the report and help formulate the decision. Lay representation on regulatory committees is becoming increasingly common as such decisions are not purely technical and scientific – they involve value judgements. Regulatory decisions are overseen and sometimes directly made by politicians who are not necessarily bound by the scientific advice they receive.

The following is a suggested approach or framework for making decisions in drug safety (i.e. a structured list of the issues that should be taken into account):

1 What is the nature of problem?
2 What is the evidence of benefit?
3 What is the evidence for risk?
4 How do we value the risks and benefits?
5 What assumptions have we made and how valid are they?
6 What areas of uncertainty remain?
7 What are the options for action?
8 What are the expected consequences of each option?

Implementation

Unless the medicine is to be withdrawn from the market, most actions which could be taken will involve a change to the marketing authorisation and product information. Occasionally the existing product information may be considered satisfactory and the problem is merely that the recommendations within it are frequently not being followed. In these circumstances 'reminder' communications may be issued, often directly by regulatory authorities and through regular bulletins by which the authorities communicate with health professionals. However, the extent to which these influence the behaviour of prescribers is unclear.

An important consideration is how quickly information needs to be made available to users (i.e. health professionals and patients). A new life-threatening ADR requires immediate communication whereas the addition of a symptom which does not appear to be associated with serious consequences (e.g. nausea) to the undesirable effects section of the product information could be part of the next routine revision of the SPC. Most issues come between these two extremes and a judgement needs to be made about the speed of action and the most appropriate method of communication.

An issue which is topical at the present time is about communication of signals to users. In the past, unconfirmed signals have rarely been actively communicated outside pharmacovigilance circles because of the uncertainty involved and because it is often difficult to make clear recommendations. However, expectations are changing and appearing to 'sit' on potentially worrying information which then leaks out may damage confidence in the system and lead to perceptions that the data are worse than is really the case. In an important recent example, the WHO Monitoring Centre published in the literature a signal of approximately ten-fold disproportionate ADR reporting identified from their spontaneous database related to statins and amyotrophic lateral sclerosis (a life-threatening neurological condition) despite much uncertainty about cause and effect. This was picked up and covered by lay media but, despite the very wide use of statins, it did not appear to create a major 'scare'. It is likely that information about signals will increasingly be actively communicated in the future.

Communication

Principles

Communication is a vital stage in the pharmacovigiwance process but one that is hard to get right, particularly if there is an urgent need to act. The oral contraceptive example discussed in Chapter 1 has led to much more attention to this aspect and agreement about the principles involved.

The main requirements for a successful drug safety communication are that it is accurate, balanced, open, understandable and targeted. These can be recalled by the mnemonic 'ABOUT':

Key requirements for a successful drug safety communication (ABOUT)

Requirement	Comments
Accurate	Are the facts and numbers correct? Is all the information which the reader needs to know included?
Balanced	Have both risks and benefits been considered? Is the overall message right?
Open	Is the communication completely honest about the hazard without any attempt to hide or minimise it?
Understandable	Should be as straightforward as possible – the reader is more likely to respond appropriately if the message is simple and clear.
Targeted	This involves considering who is the intended audience and their specific information needs.

Practicalities

The ABOUT criteria are considerations which can be used to formulate the process of developing a communication. A draft should be tested against these requirements by a review process which includes both individuals who are experts in the field and those who are generalists. Communications intended for patients should be written in plain language and reviewed by lay people. In the multi-cultural and diverse world-marketplace, making information available in the appropriate languages represents a growing challenge. In urgent situations it is vital to spend enough of the time which is available ensuring that these requirements are met.

It is particularly important in any communication about drug safety to ensure that essential information is clearly conveyed and not obscured by other less important information. The key facts and recommendations must be worded unambiguously and should be placed in a prominent early position, with use of highlighting. It is vital that the level of the risk is made very clear by expressing it in absolute rather than relative terms.

The following represents a basic model for any drug safety communication, whether it is to be targeted at health professionals or at a lay audience (e.g. the general media):

Basic model for a drug safety communication

Short heading which includes the drug and hazard

---

1 Nature of the problem: drug, hazard, precipitating factor(s)
2 Summary of the evidence for the hazard
3 What is being done: for example reviewing, investigating, new studies, changing labelling and so on
4 What are the implications for (a) health professionals (b) patients?
5 Overall balanced view of risks and benefits
6 Where to get further information/contact details

Information sent to health professionals should be clearly labelled 'Important safety information' and, if appropriate, 'Urgent'. It is also useful to prepare answers to 'Frequently asked questions' and these are often placed on relevant websites.

The role of the media in drug safety will be considered further in Chapter 7.

Measuring success

Measuring the success of actions taken to minimise risk is an important step in the overall process, but one that is often overlooked or poorly done. Broadly, the possible methods of evaluating the effectiveness of actions taken are as follows:

- **Testing the effectiveness of the communications** – have they been received and understood (e.g. using market research techniques)?
- **Analysing the effect on prescribing** – the extent to which prescribing habits are modified and are consistent with revised recommendations in product information (e.g. using longitudinal patient databases).
- **Monitoring spontaneously reported cases** to see whether serious cases continue to be reported. This may be difficult to interpret because of publicity bias but it can be useful to see, for example, whether any of the reported cases reflect contraindicated use.

- **Observation/formal study of prescribing and events** – has the action resulted in reduced morbidity/mortality from the ADR in practice? This will require use of a longitudinal patient databases or an epidemiological study and is perhaps an ideal but is the least frequently undertaken of these activities.

Crisis management

Every drug safety issue is different and an important step in dealing with one is to determine the level of urgency in using the principles discussed in Chapter 4 (broadly, the public health impact taking into account the absolute frequency of the hazard, number of users and seriousness). Major, newly identified hazards result in a need to re-evaluate the overall risk–benefit balance. The highest level of urgency occurs when new evidence emerges suggesting that the risks of a medicine may outweigh the benefits, either for all users or in specific circumstances (e.g. a particular indication). Thus, a potential or defined need to withdraw a drug on safety grounds is inevitably a crisis situation for those involved in its management. In these circumstances, any delay may result in damage to patients and reasonable haste is necessary.

Crisis management in drug safety is not fundamentally different to dealing with other types of crisis. A standard operating procedure for crisis management needs to be in place beforehand defining:
- What will be considered a crisis
- Composition of the crisis team and responsibilities
- Stakeholders and need for interactions with them

The first task of the crisis team is to draw up a specific crisis management plan which will define the following:
- Key objectives
- Expected timelines (likely to be days to a few weeks at most)
- Resources required
- Responsibilities

The key tasks for the drug safety crisis team are likely to be the following:
- Evaluation of the evidence
- Decision-making
- Practical arrangements for implementation
- Developing the external communication materials

Progress towards the objectives needs to be reviewed daily and effective internal communication is vital. Because a regulatory authority or company needs to deal with a crisis does not mean that routine work and other obligations can be ignored. Personnel who continue to deal with routine work should ideally be kept entirely separate from the crisis team.

Conclusion

This chapter has considered the process of pharmacovigilance from signal of possible hazard through to remedial action. The outlined principles apply to both pharmaceutical companies and regulatory authorities. Both parties should be involved in all stages of the process, have access to all the relevant data and communicate developments promptly to each other. Chapter 5 will consider how companies and regulators should interact to ensure that the process is appropriately applied.

CHAPTER 5

Regulatory aspects of pharmacovigilance

Introduction

As discussed in Chapter 1, the need for medicines regulation and pharmacovigilance became widely recognised in the 1960s as a consequence of thalidomide. The role of regulatory authorities is a public health function and their tasks are to protect the public health and to promote safe and effective use of medicines. In general terms, these activities are also in the interests of pharmaceutical companies but they have an additional, commercial driver – the needs to recoup investments in products and to satisfy shareholders. Since health and financial drivers may, in relation to specific issues, conflict, the authorities have compulsory powers to act on grounds of safety. However, these powers are only used when essential – most of the time regulatory authorities will seek and gain voluntary agreement from companies for the necessary measures.

Legally, both the authorities and manufacturers are responsible for the safety of medicinal products. In the European Union (EU), both parties are obliged to operate pharmacovigilance systems, to exchange data and, where necessary, to take appropriate action to protect patients. The responsibilities of the authorities cover all medicinal products – and there are many thousands of them. Therefore, in practice, they have to focus particularly on issues which are the most important for public health. Since the early post-marketing phase is invariably a period of considerable uncertainty about safety and when important new hazards are most likely to be identified, much of their attention is concentrated on newer drugs.

An Introduction to Pharmacovigilance. By Patrick Waller.
Published 2010 by Blackwell Publishing, ISBN: 978-1-4051-9471-6.

In this chapter 'regulation' will be considered from both sides of the fence. The regulatory obligations of pharmaceutical companies are extensively laid out in legislation and guidelines but it is important to appreciate that merely meeting these obligations does not ensure the safety of medicinal products. Rather, they should be seen as an essential baseline from which an acceptable safety standard can potentially be achieved. Recently it has been formally recognised that the whole process has been inherently too passive, that more and better post-authorisation safety studies are needed, and that proper planning is required if adequate safety knowledge is to be gained. This has led to the introduction of risk management planning to underpin the whole process.

Legislation and guidelines

Despite ongoing attempts at international harmonisation (see Chapter 6), legislative requirements for the regulation of medicines differ considerably around the world. In this section I shall focus solely on the EU. In the EU, most medicines legislation is underpinned by guidance which is there to give advice on how best to comply with the law. Following guidelines is generally a good practice but it may not always be possible or appropriate. Guidelines are much more easily amended than legislation and tend to increase in size as issues of interpretation arise and are addressed.

Key elements of European legislation
EU medicines legislation has two broad aims – protection of public health and the creation of a single market for pharmaceuticals. EU legislation is initially proposed by the European Commission, goes through consultative and political processes and emerges via the European Parliament to be put into force by the Commission. In principle, if there is an apparent conflict with any national legislation, EU law takes precedence. However, this does not necessarily mean that national authorities cannot enforce additional requirements in their own territory.

The legislation underpinning the centralised system of authorisation (i.e. one licence valid throughout the EU) is in the form of a Regulation – number 2309/93 (the latter number reflecting that it was originally made in 1993). This is directly effective in all Member States. Most of the other EU legislation is contained in a single Directive – 2001/83 – this obliges Member States to implement national laws having specified effects. Confusingly, the numbering order here is reversed and the year this came into force was 2001. However, there were no major changes made at that time – all that happened was that many previous Directives, going back as far as 1965, were brought together in one place. Both the Regulation and Directive alluded to above have specific sections on pharmacovigilance. These are:

- Regulation 2309/93: articles 19–26
- Directive 2001/83, Title IX, articles 101–108

When required, regulatory action is taken through the marketing authorisation. The options available are suspension, revocation or variation. These powers are specified in article 117 of Directive 2001/83 (note that this is not part of the title on pharmacovigilance). Section (c) of article 117 – an unfavourable risk-benefit balance – is the most usual ground for suspension or revocation. The former is temporary and usually put in place as a matter of urgency; the latter leads to permanent removal of the product and the decision is taken over longer time scale during which the Marketing Authorisation (MA) holder can appeal. As discussed in Chapter 4, variation of the authorisation is the most common mechanism for dealing with pharmacovigilance issues and, if urgent, there is a mechanism for making safety restrictions within 24 hours. Both the authorities and companies can initiate such restrictions.

Aside from the above legislation, the Directive covering clinical trials – 2001/20 – is relevant in relation to pharmacovigilance for investigational drugs.

The most important principles currently specified in the EU legislation may be summarised as follows:

- Pharmacovigilance is based on existing national systems
- The European Medicines Agency (EMEA) is responsible for co-ordination
- Member States are responsible for conducting pharmacovigilance in their own territories
- The common forum is the Pharmacovigilance Working Party of the Committee for Human Medicinal Products (CHMP)
- MA holders have defined responsibilities (see below)

Guidelines

Most of the EU guidance relevant to pharmacovigilance can be found in Volume 9A of the Rules Governing Medicinal Products which was issued in January 2007. This is in four parts preceded by an introduction which summarises the legal basis of the system and the roles of the various parties. The four parts are as follows:

Part I: Guidelines for Marketing Authorisation holders
Part II: Guidelines for competent authorities
Part III: Guidelines on electronic exchange of information
Part IV: Guidelines on communication

The most extensive part of Volume 9A is the first, i.e. the guidelines for MA holders. It is in eight parts, as follows:

1 General principles
2 Pharmacovigilance system requirements, monitoring of compliance and inspections
3 Risk management systems
4 Expedited reporting of individual cases
5 Reporting requirements in special situations
6 Periodic safety update reports
7 Company-sponsored post-authorisation studies
8 Overall pharmacovigilance evaluation and safety-related regulatory action

The second and third parts were largely new at the last revision, reflecting greater regulatory oversight of company systems through inspection and the introduction of risk management plans, both of which are quite recent developments.

Other documents which are relevant to pharmacovigilance include guidelines on the Summary of Product Characteristics and Package Inserts (in Volume 2 of the Rules Governing Medicinal Products), and, for investigational drugs, clinical trial guidelines (Volume 10 of the Rules Governing Medicinal Products, Chapter II).

Regulatory pharmacovigilance systems

Broadly, there are two functions to pharmacovigilance from the perspective of a regulator – (1) the protection of public health by measures to prevent serious ADRs and (2) regulation of the industry. Medicines regulatory authorities do not regulate health professionals and prescribers who are able to use medicines outside the terms of the authorisation (and unlicensed medicines) on their own responsibility.

In terms of protecting public health, regulators are active at every stage of the pharmacovigilance process described in Chapter 4. In particular, they are concerned to ensure that signals are identified as rapidly as possible and appropriately managed. They will also want to be sure that the actions taken are appropriate and communicated adequately.

In terms of regulating industry, the principal issue is one of compliance with the legal requirements. Formal monitoring of industry compliance with pharmacovigilance obligations through inspections is a fairly recent development. These inspections may be undertaken routinely or if at any time the authorities have a reason to believe there may be non-compliance. There is a three-level approach to dealing with non-compliance. Relatively minor transgressions may be dealt with by educative measures or, in more serious cases, warnings may be issued. In very serious or persistent cases, prosecution may be undertaken against the marketing authorisation holder. Offences are determined nationally but can include substantial fines and even imprisonment, with both the company and the qualified person (see below) being held responsible.

It should also be noted that regulators have obligations towards industry, in particular the timely transmission of reports which they receive from health professionals to the MA holder.

Obligations of pharmaceutical companies

Broadly, the pharmacovigilance obligations of companies may be summarised as follows:
- To operate a pharmacovigilance system with documented procedures
- To nominate a qualified person for pharmacovigilance
- ADR reporting
- Periodic safety update reporting
- To inform regulatory authorities of any information which may change the risk/benefit balance
- To respond to requests for information from regulatory authorities
- To manage and minimise risk(s) with their medicines

Company pharmacovigilance systems

The qualified person for pharmacovigilance takes personal responsibility for organisation and management of the pharmacovigilance system within the company. He or she needs to be continuously available and therefore most large companies also nominate a deputy. It is essential that adequately documented procedures are put in place and that a quality management system approach is adopted.

Effective pharmacovigilance requires a properly functioning database containing accurate and up-to-date data. All personnel within the department must be appropriately trained. General system compliance with these principles is now monitored by regulatory authorities through inspections, as discussed above. Next, I will consider in a little more detail, the principal activities undertaken by company pharmacovigilance departments, i.e. ADR reporting, periodic safety update reporting and post-authorisation safety studies.

ADR reporting

I have described the principles of spontaneous ADR reporting in Chapter 3 and how the data are used in the pharmacovigilance process in Chapter 4. It should be self-evident that the purpose of company ADR reporting obligations is to ensure that regulators have prompt access to reports which are submitted directly to companies. This has led to the concept of the 'expedited' report – in essence this is a report of a serious suspected ADR and the obligation is to submit to the authorities within 15 calendar days of receipt. Non-serious reports are not submitted individually but should be included in periodic safety update reports (see below). In the EU, reporting electronically and the use of the MedDRA for coding has recently become mandatory.

There are two other important principles for companies. The first is that serious reports should be followed-up and the information gleaned also reported within 15 days. Secondly, companies should proactively search the medical literature to identify published case reports of adverse reactions to their drugs. Assuming they are considered serious, these should also be submitted as expedited reports.

Prior to authorisation, in relation to products being investigated in clinical trials, ADR reporting requirements are different. The key principles here are that *serious and unexpected* (as defined by absence from the investigator's brochure) suspected ADRs SUSARs should be expedited, and that such reports should be unblinded for this purpose. Steps should be taken to ensure that personnel directly involved in the trial remain blinded. Companies are required to submit SUSARs both to regulatory authorities and the ethics committee(s) that approved the trial. They must also ensure that all investigators are kept informed about SUSARs so as to meet the key objective of protecting the safety of trial subjects.

The practice of ADR reporting by companies has many complexities that I have not discussed and which are best learned on-the-job through use of the available detailed regulatory guidelines. However, if the above principles are followed and cases of doubt are discussed with the authorities, you are unlikely to go far wrong.

Periodic safety update reporting

The concept of, and format for, periodic safety update reporting was developed in the early 1990s by a Council for the Organisation of Medical Sciences (CIOMS) working group (see Chapter 6) and rapidly implemented into legislation in many parts of the world. The objective of producing Periodic Safety Update Reports (PSURs) is to facilitate regular, systematic review of the *global* safety data available to the manufacturer of marketed products. The goal of such review is to identify any change in the safety profile of the product which might require further investigation or action.

Production of PSURs starts when a drug is first approved for marketing anywhere in the world (the 'international birth date' or IBD) and, initially, reports are produced on a six-monthly basis. The period covered becomes longer once the drug is established in the market but precise requirements have varied over time and between countries. PSURs are not cumulative documents – they each cover a defined period of time starting either at the IBD or when data for the previous report were 'locked'.

The contents and structure of a PSUR may be summarised as follows:

- Executive summary
- Introduction/scope of the report
- Worldwide marketing authorisation status
- Actions taken for safety reasons and changes to core safety information
- Patient exposure data
- Individual case histories (as 'line listings' and tabulations)
- Information from formal studies
- Overall safety evaluation
- Important information received after the data lock point

The 'Reference' or 'Core' Safety Information is also included, often as an appendix – this is a minimum standard of information which is considered essential for safe use and will be included in all product information worldwide.

A key section of the PSUR is the overall safety evaluation. This is where any important newly identified or ongoing safety issues are identified and proposals made to address them.

PSURs are routinely submitted to, and reviewed by, regulatory authorities around the world. Meeting all their requirements is complex and resource-intensive, despite a fair degree of harmonisation. At present, the requirements for PSURs cover all authorised products for the duration of their marketed life. A format for safety update reporting in relation to investigational drugs in development [the Development Safety Update Report (DSUR)] has been proposed by CIOMS (see Chapter 6) and changes to regulatory requirements for periodic reporting in relation to investigational drugs are likely to follow.

Post-authorisation safety studies

Companies started to conduct these studies in the 1980s, but in the early days they were often seen as covert marketing exercises intended to promote use of a new medicine. Of course, it is impossible to study safety in ordinary practice if a drug is little used but nevertheless it is important that post-marketing studies have clear safety objectives and do not interfere with prescribing practice. The emergence of databases such as the General Practice Research Database in the UK has lessened the need for 'field' studies which start by recruiting prescribing doctors and build up a cohort of users. From a scientific point of view, single cohort studies based on use of a particular drug are often of limited value. They may measure the frequency of a particular event but they do not provide any indication of the expected or background frequency, meaning that judgement of causality can only be made from the individual cases. This problem is best addressed by including a comparison cohort of patients using an alternative treatment.

Another frequent limitation of post-authorisation studies is the sample size. Historically, 10,000 patients has often been a fairly arbitrary target for a drug which is likely to be widely used – this is based on the notion that it is about one order of magnitude more than the average number of patients studied in clinical trials. In terms of studying ADRs, which are rare or very rare, this will mean that there are only likely to be a few or possibly no cases observed in the study.

In general, such studies will measure events rather than suspected ADRs but any serious events which are suspected by investigators to be drug-related should be submitted to regulatory authorities as an expedited report. Regulatory guidelines indicate that companies planning such studies should submit a protocol for review and provide data from the study in the form of interim and final reports. In practice, such interactions are now likely to be tied in with a risk management plan in most instances (see below).

Risk management planning

In recent years considerable efforts have been made by regulatory authorities and companies to improve existing systems of risk management. In the past, the pharmacovigilance process has often lacked a clear starting point and an active plan to gain further safety knowledge and minimise risks. It has now been recognised that there is a need to focus more on safety rather than harm and to actively plan to demonstrate the safety of newly authorised products. An important and fairly new development introduced in 2005 which addresses these points is Risk Management Planning. A risk management plan (RMP) may contain three sections:

• Safety specification
• Pharmacovigilance plan
• Risk minimisation plan

The purpose of the safety specification is to explicitly consider the level of safety that has been demonstrated so far. It should identify what is and *is not* yet known about safety and the latter (i.e. what is not known) should be a major driver of the pharmacovigilance plan. The purpose of that plan is essentially to attempt to find out what is not yet known, largely because of the limitations of clinical trials. Risk minimisation plans are not invariably required – essentially they are needed when there are known or potential risks which cannot simply be managed through routine measures contained in the product information.

Until recently, post-marketing safety activities in pharmaceutical companies have mainly revolved around satisfying the regulatory requirements outlined above, i.e. spontaneous reporting and periodic safety update reports. Whilst these are all important, they do not in themselves ensure that medicines are safe and often they do little to demonstrate safety. They may also encourage a tendency towards focusing on bureaucratic requirements rather than public health. Since it is impossible to know that a medicine is acceptably safe until it has been used in ordinary practice, it is reasonable to argue that demonstrating safety should be a key goal post-marketing and therefore logical that it is necessary to plan how to achieve it.

In the EU, submission of an RMP with an application for marketing authorisation is now required for all new active substances and for changes to existing authorisations which are likely to significantly extend usage of the product. Plans may also be requested by the authorities at a later stage if an important new safety issue emerges. Such plans are generally targeted to a large degree at the relevant hazard.

In the next three sections I shall consider the key principles underpinning each part of the plan.

Safety specification

Any new medicine which is to be authorised can be considered to have a level of safety which, in relation to its potential benefits and the disease being treated, is provisionally acceptable. The safety specification should document the basis of this judgement under the five broad headings set out below. Note that these are not in the order given in EU guidelines but a good starting point conceptually is to consider the disease which will be treated and the characteristics of the target population.

1 Epidemiology of the indication(s)

This should include the descriptive epidemiology of the disease indication(s), i.e. incidence, prevalence and demographic considerations, prognosis, likely co-morbidity and co-prescribing, plus medical events associated with the indication which could be mistaken for ADRs. Such information will be helpful for setting spontaneous ADR reports in context.

2 Extent of current clinical safety experience

This can be summarised in the form of graphs or tabulations with calculations of the resultant statistical power to detect adverse reactions according to duration of treatment and potential latency (i.e. time to onset), based on the following information:

- Overall numbers of patients studied for various durations of treatment and lengths of follow-up in all pre-marketing trials.
- Numbers of patients in different sub-groups split by age, gender, dose and other characteristics relevant to the disease being treated (presented by duration of treatment and length of follow-up). Both overall numbers and sub-groups are best shown graphically using plots of exposure over time (Figure 5.1).

3 Confirmed adverse reactions

The main focus here should be on ADRs identified in clinical trials described and quantified by system organ class based on statistically

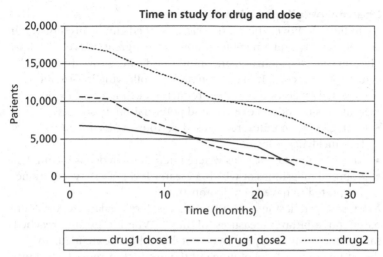

Figure 5.1 Schematic Plot of drug exposure vs time

significant differences (at the 5% level) seen between treated and control groups. This may be best presented as absolute excess risks with 95% confidence intervals.

4 Signals of potential adverse reactions

These might include the following:

- Serious events which are not statistically significantly different between groups in clinical trials but which constitute potential signals requiring further evaluation based on a relative risk of at least 2 or at least one case that was thought to be drug-related (either by the investigator or the company following a formal causality assessment).
- Unconfirmed signals of potential toxicity found in pre-clinical data.

5 Areas of safety knowledge that are incomplete

The main areas to be considered here are:

- Populations not studied in clinical trials (especially if these are not to be absolute contraindications) or where experience is limited (e.g. children).
- Rare ADRs not yet observed with the drug but which are recognised to occur with other drugs in the class or which are possible based on knowledge of the molecular structure.
- Consideration of the potential for safety concerns based on inappropriate use.

Pharmacovigilance plan

As indicated above, the marketing of a medicine represents both an opportunity and a need to demonstrate a greater level of safety. The pharmacovigilance plan should indicate how this will be achieved in practice. It might contain the following information:

- Expected levels of use of the product over time (worldwide)
- Strategies to address existing and potential safety signals
- Strategies to monitor recognised serious ADRs to ensure that their incidence is low
- Strategies to address areas where safety knowledge is incomplete
- Proposed milestones at which a greater level of safety experience is expected to have been demonstrated

Most safety milestones (e.g. periodic safety update reports) are based on arbitrary measures of time. When they are reached, safety knowledge may or may not have been extended, in part depending on the level of usage of the product. A more logical way of defining milestones is to base them on levels of exposure. They can be derived using the expected level of use, taking into account power calculations indicating the known level of safety at authorisation. Milestones are thus reached when a specified number of patients had been studied (possibly for a specified length of time), or when particular safety studies are complete.

Risk minimisation plans

These are required when product information alone is considered to provide insufficient safeguards against known or serious potential hazards. The measures contained within them vary from general education (e.g. dear health professional letters) through specific training of users in safe administration to restrictions on use-linked documentation of safe practice (e.g. ensuring that users of clozapine actually have acceptable white cell counts before a further prescription can be dispensed). Whatever level of activity is envisioned, good communication (as outlined in Chapter 4) is essential and it is important to consider and test the feasibility of the proposed measures. The most common form of activity is promotion of safe use and it is important that this is not confused with mere promotion of use. Regulators generally expect there to be clear daylight between the two activities and are unlikely to accept company representatives as a vehicle for delivery of risk minimisation measures.

As discussed in Chapter 4, the final step in the whole process of pharmacovigilance is to assess the extent to which risk minimisation is successful and if, necessary, to refine or change the measures. This is something that, in the past, has generally not been done well or at all. A lot can be learned from studies of drug utilisation and in particular from studying the characteristics of users and how a medicine is used. It is relatively easy, for example, to use a prescription database to examine concomitant use of interacting drugs (which might perhaps be contraindicated). Ideally, we would like to measure hard outcomes – i.e. to know that adverse reactions are being prevented by the measures put in place. Certainly, monitoring spontaneous ADR reports is normally insufficient for the purpose and this objective requires further research to develop the necessary tools.

Conclusion

In this chapter, I have outlined the principles underpinning pharmacovigilance and regulation focusing on the EU. Much of what I have described has been developed in part through wider international co-operation. How and why this has happened and the roles of the relevant bodies will be described in the next chapter.

CHAPTER 6
International collaboration

Introduction

There are many potential reasons for apparent international variations in the safety of medicines. The population in which a drug is used might be different in terms of ethnicity, demographic factors or the indication(s). The need for a drug and way in which a drug is used might be different (e.g. in terms of dose or monitoring), as might be perceptions of risks and benefits in relation to alternative treatments. Despite the legitimacy of such reasons, historical variations in safety recommendations and practice have undoubtedly exceeded what can be explained by them. There are many examples of drugs withdrawn or restricted in one part of the word and available in another. Such national variations often reflect uncertainty in the relevant data and differing views of experts who advise regulatory authorities on safety. Until there is less scope for debate about safety data, they are likely to continue.

International collaboration in pharmacovigilance has undoubtedly advanced greatly in recent years as communication has improved and regulatory authorities around the world have increasingly engaged in dialogue. In recent years, the EU system has addressed many of the kind of differences alluded to above across the Member States through systems of centralisation and arbitration.

Marketing pharmaceuticals is generally a global business and much impetus has come from the industry towards international harmonisation of standards. In this respect, considerable progress has been made in the past two decades, largely through the auspices of the three organisations – the World Health Organisation, the Council for the Organisation of Medical Sciences and the International Conference on Harmonisation. The activities and

An Introduction to Pharmacovigilance. By Patrick Waller.
Published 2010 by Blackwell Publishing, ISBN: 978-1-4051-9471-6.

achievements of each in relation to pharmacovigilance are discussed in this chapter.

World Health Organisation (WHO)

The WHO's international collaborative programme on drug safety was originally set up in 1968. Their monitoring centre is now based in Uppsala, Sweden. The main activities of the centre are as follows:

- Co-ordinating the WHO Programme for International Drug Monitoring
- Collecting, assessing and communicating information from member countries about the benefits and risks of drugs
- Collaborating with member countries in the development and practice of pharmacovigilance
- Alerting regulatory authorities of member countries about potential drug safety problems.

At the time of writing, there were 84 national schemes which collaborate with the programme and provide their spontaneous ADR reports to the WHO at least four times per year. The data are entered onto a database which is an international reference source accessible to national authorities and pharmaceutical companies. By mid-2008 this database held around 3.7 million case reports.

For analysis, the WHO centre uses a data-mining approach (see Chapter 4) supported by clinical assessment provided by a panel of reviewers in order to identify signals of new adverse reactions. Information is exchanged between WHO and the national centres electronically through 'Vigimed'. The Uppsala Monitoring Centre also publishes periodic newsletters and is responsible for managing the WHO Drug Dictionary and the WHO Adverse Reaction Terminology (WHOART). The former is a widely used international standard but the latter has now largely been superseded by the MedDRA. The Centre also provides training and support to countries establishing pharmacovigilance systems, particularly in the developing world. There is an annual meeting of representatives of collaborating centres at which scientific and organisational matters are discussed.

Council for the Organisation of Medical Sciences (CIOMS)

The CIOMS is based in Geneva and operates under the WHO umbrella. It has served as a forum for discussions between regulators and industry on a variety of pharmacovigilance topics since the late 1980s. Over the years, reports from CIOMS working groups have been highly influential in shaping legislation and guidelines around the world. To date, there have been eight formal CIOMS working groups – the topics and broad vision of each group are summarised below:

CIOMS I: International reporting of ADRs (1990)

Before the mid-1980s, reporting requirements to regulatory authorities related almost entirely to domestic ADR reports, i.e. those occurring on national territory. Some countries then started to introduce requirements for submission of 'foreign' reports. This working group was convened to discuss the principles of what should be reported and how. The key output was that such reports should be of suspected reactions which were both serious **and** unexpected (i.e. unlabelled). The group also proposed that 15 days was the appropriate maximum time frame for submission and developing a reporting form – the 'CIOMS form' which became the international standard. In 1995 the working group reconvened (known as CIOMS Ia) and made proposals for the data elements to be included in electronic transmission of reports.

CIOMS II: International reporting of periodic safety update summaries (1992)

This report made the original proposals for the format and content of PSURs. Since 1992, requirements for PSURs have been widely implemented as a regulatory requirement (see Chapter 5) and a harmonised guideline has been adopted through the International Conference on Harmonisation (see below).

CIOMS III: Guidelines for preparing core clinical-safety information on drugs (1995)

This report addressed the problem of variations in safety labelling around the world by proposing that manufacturers should develop a 'core data sheet' that contains all the relevant safety information which needs to be included in all countries where the drug is marketed. This is effectively a minimum standard – additional information may be included in some countries – and it also serves as the basis for deciding whether or not a specific adverse reaction is 'listed' (i.e. expected) or not. The report made specific recommendations as to what should be included in core safety information, and when and how it should be included.

CIOMS IV: Benefit-risk balance for marketed drugs – evaluating safety signals (1998)

This report proposes a standard format and content for a benefit-risk evaluation report and also lays down the principles for good decision-making practices. The proposed structure of the report is as follows:

1 Introduction
2 Benefit evaluation
3 Risk evaluation
4 Benefit-risk evaluation
5 Options analysis

CIOMS V: Current challenges in pharmacovigilance – pragmatic approaches (2001)

This report is about good case management and reporting practices, both in terms of individual cases and summaries. It includes almost 20 pages of detailed and specific recommendations. The general thrust of the report is that, despite a lot of progress towards harmonisation, there is much that remains inefficient and that the ultimate goal should be a single, global shared data set.

CIOMS VI: Management of safety information from clinical trials (2005)

The aim of this report was to enhance awareness of the ethical and technical issues associated with safety in clinical trials. It proposes a systematic approach to managing safety during clinical development and is wide-ranging, covering, e.g., ethical issues, statistical approaches to identifying risks and communication of safety information from clinical trials.

CIOMS VII: The Development Safety Update Report (DSUR) – harmonising the format and content for periodic safety reporting during clinical trials (2006)

This report proposes the content and format for a DSUR – a means of regular and timely review, appraisal and communication of safety information during the clinical development of drugs. The working group envisions that, in the future, the DSUR and PSUR could be integrated into a single harmonised safety report that would cover a product throughout its lifecycle.

CIOMS VIII: Application of signal detection in pharmacovigilance

This working group is focused on signal detection and management, and their report is expected to be published soon.

Other activities of CIOMS

In addition to the projects discussed above, there are ongoing CIOMS working groups addressing the following issues:

- Vaccine pharmacovigilance
- Pharmacogenetics
- Drug development research and pharmacovigilance in resource-poor countries

CIOMS has also been involved in developing definitions of ADR terms and the rational use of standardised MedDRA queries, and in ethical guidelines for epidemiological studies.

International Conference on Harmonisation

The International Conference on Harmonisation (ICH) is a more formal group than CIOMS with a wider remit for harmonisation across the drug development process. It has also been influential in shaping current regulatory requirements relating to pharmacovigilance. ICH involves representatives from regulators and industry and is tripartite in terms of regions, covering the EU, USA and Japan. There are also various observers, e.g. from the WHO. The main purpose is to harmonise existing guidelines from the three regions related to development and registration of medicines.

ICH guidelines have a five-step development process, as follows:

- Step 1 – Preliminary discussion by relevant experts and production of a draft
- Step 2 – The draft is considered and 'signed-off' by the Steering Committee
- Step 3 – Wider consultation and revision
- Step 4 – Final 'sign off' by the Steering Committee
- Step 5 – Implementation into the relevant legislation and guidelines

In principle, the authorities in each territory are committed to implementing ICH, guidelines although, in practice, the timing and extent of implementation have been variable.

There are four broad categories of ICH guideline, as follows:

- Quality (Q)

- Safety (S)
- Efficacy (E)
- Multidisciplinary (M)

In this context, 'Safety' means pre-clinical guidelines and the clinical safety guidelines have been classified under efficacy. In relation to pharmacovigilance, the key ICH guidelines and dates at which they were implemented are:

- E2A: Definitions and Standards for Expedited Reporting (1994)
- E2B: Data Elements for Electronic transmission of Individual Case Safety Reports (1997)
- E2C: Periodic Safety Update Reports for Marketed Drugs (1996)
- E2D: Post-approval Safety Data Management (2003)
- E2E: Pharmacovigilance Planning (2005)

The MedDRA was originally developed through the ICH process (M1) and is now maintained by a Maintenance and Support Service Organisation (MSSO).

Conclusion

The harmonisation activities described above can be regarded as 'work in progress'. Perhaps the most glaring remaining hole is the absence of an overall international standard for pharmacovigilance (i.e. Good Pharmacovigilance Practice). Developing such a standard is likely to prove a major challenge but is vital for the future of discipline (see Chapter 8).

CHAPTER 7
Ethical and societal considerations

Introduction

So far, I have focused on the discipline of pharmacovigilance as it is practised at the industry/regulator interface. This chapter considers wider societal aspects of the safety of medicines, starting by identifying the main stakeholders and their perspectives. There is an important ethical dimension to pharmacovigilance – medicines are supposed to be beneficial and yet we know that harms will occur despite best efforts to prevent them. In the past, much information about the safety of medicines has remained cocooned between companies and regulators. Some steps to improve transparency have been made both in terms of process and access to the relevant data. Potential conflicts of interest abound and need to be handled appropriately. Public confidence in the system is not high and there are fierce critics who believe that regulators and industry are too cosy, and that patient's interests do not always come first. The media watch over from a distance waiting for something interesting to happen.

Stakeholders and their perspectives

The most important stakeholders in pharmacovigilance are patients who use medicines – this is, after all, why the discipline exists. Health professionals are also 'users' of the medicines they prescribe and both probably have similar expectations of the process. Broadly speaking, users of medicines expect them to have been adequately tested, to be 'safe' in the sense that serious harms are unlikely to occur and to be provided with appropriate and understandable

An Introduction to Pharmacovigilance. By Patrick Waller.
Published 2010 by Blackwell Publishing, ISBN: 978-1-4051-9471-6.

information about their use. These are in essence the goals of the regulatory process but due to limitations that largely have a scientific basis there is probably a gap between expectation and reality. Patients know that 'side-effects' can occur with medicines but generally perceive these as likely to be transient or reversible and non-serious. When a life-threatening reaction occurs with a treatment given for a relatively trivial indication they are shocked. The prescribing doctor is too since he/she has unintentionally broken one of the first rules of medicine – *primum non nocere* (first, do no harm). By contrast, personnel working in drug safety, whether they are in industry, a regulator or in academia, are unsurprised.

Nowadays, patients exist not only as individuals but in groups (i.e. patient organisations) and such bodies play an important role in educating and supporting individuals who develop chronic diseases. Generally they are more focused on access to treatments than on safety considerations and their perspective may well be that the need for and potential benefits of treatments outweigh quite major risks. Some patient groups are specifically based around the victims of particular treatments (e.g. there is still a prominent thalidomide action group in the UK) and they may be seeking to achieve recognition of a problem, regulatory measures against the drug or compensation for affected individuals.

Vaccines are a particularly sensitive area for understandable reasons – they are usually given to healthy individuals and often to children. One of the reasons for administering them as widely as possible may also be a benefit to society rather than the individual – i.e. 'herd' immunity. This raises an ethical dilemma if serious harms are possible. Perhaps for such reasons vaccines are unusual, in that some attempts to compensate victims directly (i.e. without litigation) have been made. In general, society does not compensate victims of ADRs unless they are prepared to litigate. To win they are likely to have to prove individual causation, i.e. they were personally harmed by the treatment (this may be intrinsically difficult as was discussed in Chapter 2) and possibly also that the manufacturer did not take all reasonable steps to identify and prevent such harm. Litigation about medicines is a major industry in itself and extremely good business for lawyers who may actively advertise for cases and pursue mass actions which are quite often settled out of court by companies as a means of damage limitation. Health ministers are ultimately responsible for the overall system but politicians generally avoid involvement – there is little in it for them but a potential minefield to cross.

When an unexpected major drug safety issue arises, it is good copy and likely to receive a very high profile in the media. Hindsight will be liberally applied – surely this could have been predicted or avoided – and the company and/or regulators are likely to be blamed. The plight of individual victims is highlighted, but media and public interest will generally be transient. The media see their role as to inform and entertain and vary considerably in their approach but common to all is a focus on what they perceive will attract their customers (i.e. what 'sells newspapers'). Drug safety matters will do so but some elements of the matter – e.g. uncertainties and difficult judgements – are often handled badly or ignored.

Media coverage may unnecessarily scare some people into inappropriate action but pharmacovigilance personnel should not lose sight of the potential positive power of their influence. Indeed better handling of the media should be on their agenda – it is certainly worth sitting down with more responsible sections of the media and explaining what the problem is and that they can help. Ultimately, anything that may lead to well-balanced coverage and clear, appropriate messages is worth pursuing.

In terms of trying to prevent unnecessary drug safety scares, it is worth bearing in mind recognised 'fright factors' – these are aspects of a particular risk that will tend to make most people more risk-averse. In particular, we tend to be more frightened by risks which are:

• Involuntarily taken
• Man-made
• Irreversible
• Poorly understood

Many serious ADRs will meet all of these criteria meaning that it is very easy for the public to become more scared than is appropriate and to lose sight of the balancing benefits. For example, following concerns that human insulins might be associated with unawareness of hypoglycaemia in the early 1990s, some patients stopped taking insulin altogether.

All the parties mentioned above are stakeholders in the process of pharmacovigilance, but with the exception of industry and regulators they are mostly involved when a problem has already occurred. Generally, only industry personnel, regulator and individual users (i.e. patients/health professionals) between them have the potential to prevent some specific problems occurring – the ultimate purpose of the process. Other stakeholders may influence the system or endeavour to promote change but most of the impetus for improvement tends to come from regulator/industry interface.

Ethical principles

As should be clear from above, there are many potential tensions in the drug safety system – e.g. risk vs. benefit, individual vs. population good, potential therapeutic gain from innovation vs. uncertainty. These are set in a background of commercial and political imperatives, the latter largely being the economics of healthcare. The need for an ethical approach and ethical safeguards is therefore manifest.

In terms of researching the safety of medicines in human subjects, there is an overarching code of ethical principles – The *Declaration of Helsinki* – which was originally developed under the auspices of the World Medical Association in 1964. The last significant revision was in 2000 and this is currently a fairly brief document with some 32 points. The most significant ones in the context of safety are:

* 'In medical research on human subjects, considerations related to the well-being of the human subject should take precedence over the interests of science and society'.
* 'Every medical research project involving human subjects should be preceded by careful assessment of predictable risks and burdens in comparison with foreseeable benefits to the subject or to others'.
* 'Medical research involving human subjects should only be conducted if the importance of the objective outweighs the inherent risks'.

These have an underlying theme, i.e. *individual* patient safety is paramount.

When experimental research is being conducted (i.e. there is some intervention which would not occur in ordinary practice – e.g. randomisation), informed consent is considered essential. For non-experimental research (i.e. mere observation of ordinary practice), consent of individuals is generally not required and may not be feasible. The patient's right to privacy is a key issue and individual patient data need to be anonymised and held securely. Confidentiality legislation varies considerably between countries and potential future increases in stringency may threaten the viability of epidemiological research.

One broad ethical question following from the principles of *Declaration of Helsinki* is: can the common good override individual perspectives and if so when? This is relevant, for example, to whether or not patient consent is required for ADR reporting and epidemiological research. In the past there has been some acceptance that the common good can override individual perspectives but we seem to moving in the direction of the rights of the individual being paramount. A related issue in pharmacovigilance is that risk/benefit trade-offs made at the population level usually accept that some individuals will lose out. Essentially, a judgement is being made that more good than harm will occur in the population in the full knowledge that some harms cannot be prevented.

There are various other specific ethical issues that face industry personnel and are relevant to safety. For example:

- Ethical promotion of drugs given the potential link between safety and promotion
- Public representation of data (e.g. the temptation towards suppression of unfavourable data or expert opinions)
- Drug pricing and availability, especially in the developing world, may lead to use of less safe medicines

Ethical safeguards in relation to safety

These may be considered on four levels:

Legislation and voluntary codes
Many of the issues discussed above are addressed in the framework of medicines legislation and in codes such as the *Declaration of Helsinki*. The pharmaceutical industry also has some voluntary codes, e.g. in relation to advertising practices.

Ethics committees/review boards
The role of such committees is to consider ethical aspects of specific research proposals and some lay representation is now the norm. Their key task is to review protocols and any amendments that may be necessary. The safety of trial subjects is always a major consideration.

Data monitoring committees
These are set up mostly in the context of a large randomised trial in order to protect subjects from safety hazards which might only

become evident during the course of the study. They should be run independently of the sponsor and operate separately from those involved in the day-to day operation of the trial. A Data Monitoring Committee looks at the safety data sequentially as it emerges and could recommend that the trial be stopped on safety grounds if it became clear that patients in one treatment arm were at greater risk of a serious hazard than in the other arm(s).

Publication

Much but not all medical research will eventually be published in the literature. Publication is selective (and therefore biased) depending on (1) what the results show – positive research is more likely to published than something which failed to observe a clear effect and (2) choices made by researchers and editors. Aside from the issue of non-publication (or delayed publication) of important research there is also the problem of misconduct. There are many potential types of misconduct relating to publication, the most serious of which are plagiarism, fraud or fabrication. In recent years steps have been taken to address these problems in part through the setting up of a Committee on Publication Ethics. This has drawn up guidelines intended to encourage intellectual honesty, prevent and deal with misconduct and provide advice on when research papers should be retracted.

Transparency

In the past, drug safety was, like many other processes involving regulated industry, essentially non-transparent. Users were expected to accept that behind the scenes, people were doing their best and with the right motives. The move towards greater transparency that gained impetus during the 1990s was not specific to this field but part of a wider societal desire to know more of what was going on. Governments have also seen advantages in opening up such processes in terms of public confidence in systems and in increasing the credibility of their decisions and advice. This change in approach has been greatly facilitated by developments in electronic communication. Thus general public policy on freedom of information has begun to override the potential commercial considerations that were for a long time the main putative reason for secrecy. It is now increasingly accepted that drug safety information rarely has real commercial value to competitors.

The following is a list of some of the major types of safety data which may now be freely available.

- Published scientific literature
- Warnings on specific issues
- Drug safety bulletins
- Press releases
- Public assessment reports
- Searchable ADR databases
- Clinical trial protocols and data

The ordering of the list is chronological in the sense that 50 years ago only information published in the scientific literature was available and that the others have been introduced at various time points since then. The last three are products of the last decade or so and far from universal even now. There is plenty of scope for further development – e.g. risk management plans have so far rarely been made public – and, in Europe at least, regulatory discussions are still held entirely behind closed doors, things which may change in the not too distant future.

Although the internet has largely solved issues of feasibility, there are some outstanding issues about provision of information. Timing of release of information is important since it is reasonable to be concerned that premature release before considered recommendations can be made could do more harm than good. There is also concern that complex information might be misunderstood and there is a need to improve delivery with the goal of aiding better understanding according the needs of the recipient.

Besides the information on which judgements and decisions are based, there is a need for transparency of process. In this respect the public need to know:

- Who reached the decision?
- What was the basis for the decision?
- Was the decision challenged?
- Why was another course of action not chosen?

Conflicts of interest

The realisation that we all have conflicts of interest and attempts to deal with them is a surprisingly recent phenomenon. It was only after the turn of the millennium that one of the major journals in the field introduced a clear policy in relation to the need for declaration of such conflicts. Drug safety is now a very sensitive area in this respect because difficult judgements have to be made about the risk of serious harms and these have financial consequences for the company involved. The public need to be convinced that those making the judgements are uninfluenced by such considerations and yet academic experts in the field are ubiquitously associated with, and their research is often funded by, the industry. In dealing with conflicts of interest, public credibility is the key issue.

There is general agreement that financial conflicts of interest must be disclosed and that persons with important conflicts should not influence relevant decisions. A useful categorisation of financial conflicts developed by regulators is to consider whether they are:

- Personal (consultancy fees, shares) or
- Non-personal (e.g. funding to a university department) and
- Specific (to the drug/issue at hand) or
- Non-specific (e.g. related to other drugs made by the same company).

Using such a system provides for four categories, and interests which are both personal and specific represent the highest level of conflict. These should result in exclusion of an expert from giving advice to regulators. Conversely, a non-personal, non-specific interest is at the lowest level and merely requires declaration. Such systems are necessary because, in practical terms, regulators would not have access to the necessary expertise if they simply excluded all experts who had any kind of conflict.

Other competing interests (e.g. non-financial) are also possible and systems are less well developed in dealing with them. Involvement with competitor products/companies, indirect potential conflicts via personal associations through family or work and past interests which might be considered lapsed are examples of such grey areas. It is likely that approaches to dealing with conflicts of interest will become yet more stringent in the future.

Conclusion

In this chapter I have outlined broad ethical and societal considerations which impact on pharmacovigilance. In terms of ethics, a balance is required between protecting individuals and the common good. To support system credibility, the need for transparency of drug safety information and processes is increasingly being recognised. It would be in everyone's interest if society as a whole was prepared to take more than a fleeting interest in pharmacovigilance. Ultimately drugs will become safer through moving the science forwards but this needs wider support which might be achieved if drug safety could be moved up the political agenda and there was better media coverage. Consideration could also be given to dealing more effectively with the victims of serious ADRs.

CHAPTER 8
Future directions

Introduction: current limitations

Since the thalidomide disaster more than 40 years ago, considerable strides have been made in all aspects of the risk management process for medicines. The drugs in use now are quite different; many new classes of medicine having been developed and they have turned out to be acceptably safe in practice. Nevertheless, there is little doubt that ADRs remain an important cause of morbidity and mortality in the developed world. Much of this harm remains potentially preventable and our current inability to prevent it is likely to directly reflect the limitations of existing systems. When thinking about the future of pharmacovigilance, a useful starting point is to consider the most important current limitations of the discipline. Hopefully, future developments will be targeted at overcoming at least some of them, although the challenges are considerable. Broadly these limitations might be characterised under three headings as follows:

1 *Predicting and understanding unexpected ADRs*
Presently, our ability to predict the occurrence of serious ADRs is limited in two senses:

(a) Despite thorough clinical development, unexpected and sometimes unexplainable ADRs become recognised at a fairly late stage in the process.

(b) It is often not possible to predict or understand why a particular individual experiences an ADR whilst another does not.

2 *Measuring the occurrence of ADRs*
Some ADRs – those that are common and obvious – are relatively easy to measure but most serious ADRs are not. This problem essentially reflects the limitations of the data sources we have

---

An Introduction to Pharmacovigilance. By Patrick Waller.
Published 2010 by Blackwell Publishing, ISBN: 978-1-4051-9471-6.

available. Often educated guesses have to be made about the
frequency of an ADR, who is most at risk and the applicability of
the available data to a general population of users.

3 *Preventing known ADRs*
Once an ADR is recognised and, perhaps even well-understood,
our ability to prevent it often remains imperfect for two broad
reasons:
(a) Few of the preventive tools used are 100% effective – e.g.
    monitoring liver function tests in a patient using a potentially
    hepatotoxic drug is unlikely to prevent all cases.
(b) Most of the preventive measures available are recommenda-
    tions which are imperfectly followed by clinicians and/or
    patients.

In overall terms, difficulties we have in predicting, understanding
and measuring ADRs hamper preventive efforts but, even if those
limitations could be overcome, the mechanisms to minimise as far
as possible serious ADRs would still need to be improved.

Meeting the challenges

Science

A logical approach to improving anything is to specifically target
areas of weakness. For example, it is notable that the most toxic
class of medicines, i.e. anti-cancer drugs, tend to be associated
with very few ADR reports. In the 1990s there was a particular
difficulty in studying the then new anti-HIV drug which was probably related to concerns about confidentiality and the underlying
diagnosis. In the UK a targeted reporting scheme was set up which
successfully allayed the concerns of reporters and gained much
important information about the safety of the class. Possibly the
most striking area of weakness has been in relation to children
who, until recent times, have been largely excluded from drug
development programmes and treated outside the terms of marketing authorisations. This is now being addressed through pae-
diatric development plans and pharmacovigilance is an important
element of them.

   Developments in molecular biology and genetics are expected
to have a considerable impact on pharmacovigilance within the
next few years. The nature and usage of new active substances is
changing substantially with more niche biological products and
new technologies such as gene therapy becoming available. These

provide new challenges for those involved in monitoring safety and increasingly require the use of registries in order to collect information on everyone who is exposed (see Chapter 3).

The discipline of pharmacogenetics is based on the premise that genetic markers may predict the safety of many drugs, with potential implications for their practical use. So far it has mostly been focused on genetic variations in hepatic drug metabolism. In the future, ADRs could be preventable through recording of personal pharmacogenetic profiles and development of guidance recommending use or avoidance of drugs, or tailored dosage regimens, for patients with specific genotypes.

In terms of the overall process of pharmacovigilance, several years ago a scientific model to support excellence in the discipline was proposed by Evans and myself (Figure 8.1).

The model represented a long-term vision of how pharmacovigilance could be conducted in the future and was underpinned by the following key concepts:

- Pharmacovigilance should be less focused on finding harm and more on extending knowledge of safety.
- There should be a clear starting point or 'specification' of what is already known at the time of licensing a medicine and what is required to extend safety knowledge post-authorisation.
- Complex risk-benefit decisions are amenable to, and likely to be improved by, the use of formal decision analysis.

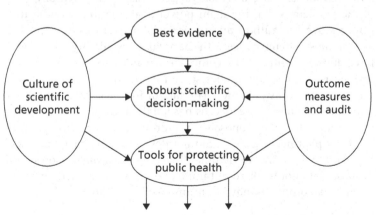

Measurable performance in terms of public health benefit

Figure 8.1 Model for excellence in pharmacovigilance.

- A new approach to provision of safety information which allows greater flexibility in presenting key messages based on multiple levels of information with access determined by user requirements.
- Flexible decision support is the most likely means of changing the behaviour of health professionals in order to promote safer use of medicines.
- There is a need to put in place outcome measures that indicate the success or failure of the process.
- Systematic audit of pharmacovigilance processes and outcomes should be developed and implemented based on agreed standards.
- Pharmacovigilance should operate in a culture of scientific development. This requires the right balance of inputs from various disciplines, a strong academic base, adequate training and resource which is dedicated to scientific strategy.

Some progress in these directions has since been made – e.g. with the development of risk management plans which include a safety specification. There are also encouraging current initiatives towards a 'culture of scientific development' in the EU with the emergence of collaborative research networks and new training programs. However, there is still quite a long way to go.

Regulation

Regulation of pharmaceuticals has traditionally been much stronger before authorisation than after it. This is understandable and to some extent appropriate but the need for stronger regulation post-authorisation is being increasingly recognised. Paradoxically, part of the problem is that the main power available to the authorities – to remove the authorisation – is too draconian to be appropriate in most circumstances. In particular, regulatory authorities have found it difficult to compel companies to conduct necessary post-authorisation studies since there is no specific legislative requirement – only guidance. The fallout from rofecoxib and other important recent safety concerns has led the European Commission to consult and make proposals on improving the legislative framework for pharmacovigilance. Similar developments have been taking place in the USA. At the time of writing, the Commission's legal proposals are not finalised but implementation is planned for 2010. Their initial proposals may be summarised as follows:

Measures to strengthen regulation
- A new pharmacovigilance committee

- Development of a *Good Vigilance Practice* standard
- An increased focus on risk management
- An obligation on companies to submit to the authorities all clinical trial data for authorised products regardless of the indication being studied
- Regulatory oversight of post-authorisation studies backed by legal powers
- Scope for better communication outputs
- Powers to limit supply to existing users of a drug (i.e. prevent new starters)

Measures to increase efficiency in industry
- Requirements for pharmacovigilance system documentation simplified through introduction of a master file
- Simplified ADR reporting requirements
- PSUR requirements to be reduced
- Primary responsibility for literature monitoring to be transferred to the regulators

Measures to increase transparency
- Introduction of a web portal for pharmacovigilance information
- Information about risk management systems to be in the public domain
- Referral procedures to be more open with public hearings

Whilst the details are still to be determined, there is wide support for the broad principles and there seems to be little doubt that post-authorisation regulation will become stronger, requirements of industry streamlined and the process more transparent.

Conclusion

In this chapter, I have tried to give a high-level glimpse of the future directions of pharmacovigilance. The next and final chapter summarises how the newcomer can deepen his or her knowledge of the subject, hopefully putting him or her in a position to contribute to meeting the challenges I have outlined.

CHAPTER 9
Learning more about pharmacovigilance

Books

There are four large textbooks that I would recommend, as follows:

Pharmacovigilance 2nd edition, 2007 (eds. Mann and Andrews)

This is a large multi-author text with 52 chapters in five sections covering (1) the basis of pharmacovigilance, (2) signal generation, (3) pharmacovigilance and selected system organ classes, (4) current key topics and (5) lessons and directions.

Pharmacoepidemiology 4th edition, 2005 (ed. Strom)

This has become the standard text on the subject. There is also an abridged, paperback version.

Stephens' Detection of New Adverse Drugs Reactions 5th edition, 2004 (eds. Talbot and Waller)

This book has broader scope than the title suggests and covers pharmacovigilance from industry, academic and regulatory perspectives. A new edition is in preparation and it might be best to wait for that.

Manual of Drug Safety and Pharmacovigilance, 2006 (ed. Cobert)

This is a very practical book with an American focus.

An Introduction to Pharmacovigilance. By Patrick Waller.
Published 2010 by Blackwell Publishing, ISBN: 978-1-4051-9471-6.

In terms of reference books about the adverse effects of drugs, the following are generally the first places to go:

Meyler's Side Effects of Drugs 15th edition, 2006 (ed. Aronson)

Authoritative and well-referenced, if this is not in the library you use then it should be.

Martindale: The Complete Drug Reference 36th edition, 2009 (ed. Sweetman)

Broader in scope than *Meyler's*, if you need to find out about any drug and its adverse effects, this is a good place to start.

Journals

Quite a few important papers in the field, including the findings of major studies, are published in the major weekly general medical journals such as the *New England Journal of Medicine, The Lancet, British Medical Journal* and *JAMA*. It is therefore a good idea to screen the contents of these titles and also the major clinical pharmacology journals. In terms of specialist journals in the field of pharmacovigilance, the two major titles, both of which appear monthly are:

- *Drug Safety*
- *Pharmacoepidemiology and Drug Safety*

The latter regularly includes a section called 'current awareness' which lists recent literature relevant to drug safety. Another journal which is very useful in that respect is *Reactions Weekly* which is primarily an alerting service based on case reports but also covers topical issues and news in the field. All these journals are available in both paper and electronic formats and access is essential for anyone working in the field.

Useful websites

The World Health Organisations' monitoring centre in Sweden (http://www.who-umc.org) is the place to go for worldwide spontaneous ADR data. The site has a global focus and much useful information besides.

The websites of major regulatory agencies are also worth visiting regularly for information about specific issues/alerts, bulletins and ADR data. In particular:

European Medicines Agency (EMEA): http://www.emea.europa.eu

US Food and Drug Administration (FDA): http://www.fda.gov

UK Medicines and Healthcare products Regulatory Agency (MHRA): http://www.mhra.gov.uk

The European Commission's website contains ready access to relevant EU legislation and guidance plus information about the proposed legislative changes discussed in Chapter 8 (http://ec.europa.eu/enterprise/pharmaceuticals/index_en.htm).

Courses

There are now a variety of options in several countries, from basic two-day courses run by the Drug Safety Research Unit in the UK (http://www.dsru.org) through to certificate, diploma and masters level. Training courses are also run by the two international societies mentioned below.

International societies

Finally, there are two relevant societies which exist to promote development of, and international collaboration in, their disciplines. Both hold major annual scientific meetings which would be well worth attending.

- International Society of Pharmacovigilance (ISoP): http://www.isoponline.org
- International Society of Pharmacoepidemiology (ISPE): http://www.pharmacoepi.org

Conclusion

The overarching messages I would like the newcomer to take away from this book are as follows:

Pharmacovigilance is..............

- A means of potentially preventing patients coming to serious harm as a result of the medicines they take in expectation of benefit through:
  - Science
  - Regulation
  - Clinical practice
- The final but vital stage of drug development: there is a need for a medicine to be shown to be acceptably safe in practice.

- A developing discipline with a global focus and plenty of scope for innovation.

One of the attractions of the field that may not be immediately obvious is that, although pharmacovigilance is a specialised subject, its application is very broad indeed. Every issue is different and there are no set recipes for dealing with the next safety concern to land on your desk.

Glossary

Below is a series of brief definitions and explanations of some of the most important terms used in this book.

Adverse drug reaction (ADR) An *unintended and noxious effect* that is attributable to a medicine when it has been given within the normal range of doses used in man (see p. 15).

Adverse event (AE) An undesirable occurrence that occurs in the context of drug treatment but which *may or may not* be causally related to a medicine (see p. 16).

Black Triangle scheme A scheme introduced in the UK in the 1980s to promote intensive surveillance of new drugs. An inverted black triangle is displayed on all product information as a reminder to health professionals to report all suspected ADRs. The period of intensive surveillance is usually at least two years (see p. 6).

Case-control study A study which starts by identifying cases of the disease of interest (in this context usually a potential ADR) and makes comparisons of their past 'exposures' (e.g. to drugs) with those of controls who did not develop the disease (see p. 39).

Cohort study A study which starts by identifying a particular population with a common characteristic (i.e. a cohort), often based on use of a specific drug and follows them forward in time until some individuals have developed the disease(s) of interest (see p. 39).

Clinical trial A formal study of a treatment conducted in patients with a specific disease indication. Such studies usually involve comparison with placebo or an alternative treatment and a randomisation process is used to determine the allocation of treatments. Ideally, they also involve blinding of patients and clinicians (i.e. they are 'double-blind') to treatment allocations. Conducting a clinical trial involves intervening in patients' treatments for research purposes and therefore informed consent from each patient and ethical committee approval are essential (see p. 31).

Disproportionality   A statistical indication of a signal in spontaneous ADR data meaning that more reports of a specific drug/ADR combination have been received than would have been expected as 'background noise' (see p. 46).

Observational study   A study in which there is no intervention in relation to the management of patients. Observational research is based on data derived from ordinary medical practice (see p. 38).

Orphan drug   A drug used in the treatment of an 'orphan', i.e. rare disease. Because development may be uneconomic, incentives to companies are provided. They are often authorised 'early' because of a lack of suitable alternative treatments and on the basis of small clinical trial programmes (see p. 24).

Periodic Safety Update Report (PSUR)   A systematic review of the *global* safety data which became available to the manufacturer of a marketed drug during a specified time period in an internationally agreed format. Submission of PSURs to regulatory authorities is a legal obligation in many countries (see p. 67).

Pharmacoepidemiology   The scientific discipline of studying drug effects in populations (see p. 38).

Pharmacogenetics   The use of genetic markers to maximise the safety and/or efficacy of drugs (see p. 91).

Pharmacovigilance   The science and activities relating to the detection, assessment, understanding and prevention of adverse effects or any other drug-related problems (this is the current definition of the World Health Organisation – see p. 2).

Post-marketing surveillance (PMS)   Safety-related activity after a product is marketed. This process includes but is not limited to spontaneous ADR reports. Pharmacovigilance activities start before a product is marketed; after marketing this term may be regarded as synonymous with pharmacovigilance and, nowadays, it is less frequently used (see p. 33).

Pre-clinical studies   Studies conducted in laboratory animals; these are normally performed before initiating a clinical trial programme (see p. 30).

Prescription-event monitoring (PEM)   A pharmacoepidemiological study in which a cohort of users of a medicine is identified from prescriptions and followed-up for a defined period (often 6–12 months) so as to identify all adverse events occurring in the early post-treatment period. The data are potentially useful for detecting signals of unexpected effects and/or to further study known or potential safety issues (see p. 40).

Risk Management Plan   A document prepared by a pharmaceutical company specifying what is and is not known about the safety of a product, what is planned to extend safety knowledge and how known risks will be minimised (see p. 69).

Seriousness   This term has a specific meaning in relation to a reported adverse reaction (or event). A case should be considered 'serious' if it meets any of the following criteria:

• Fatal outcome
• Life-threatening
• Led to or prolonged hospitalisation
• Led to long-term disability
• Congenital abnormality

In addition, it is possible for a case to be medically judged as serious even if none of the above criteria are met (see p. 4).

Side-effect   An unintended effect of a medicine (see p. 15).

Signal   An alert requiring further investigation from any available data source that a drug *may* be associated with a previously unrecognised hazard. The term is also used when there is new evidence that a known hazard *may* be quantitatively (e.g. more frequent) or qualitatively (e.g. more serious) different from what was previously known (see p. 44).

Spontaneous ADR report   A case report relating to an individual patient describing a *suspected* adverse reaction (see p. 33).

Summary of Product Characteristics   A regulatory document attached to the marketing authorisation which forms the basis of the product information made available to prescribers and patients (see p. 52-3).

Yellow Card Scheme   The UK national spontaneous ADR reporting scheme (see p. 5).

INDEX